Practical Nutrition for a Fit Life

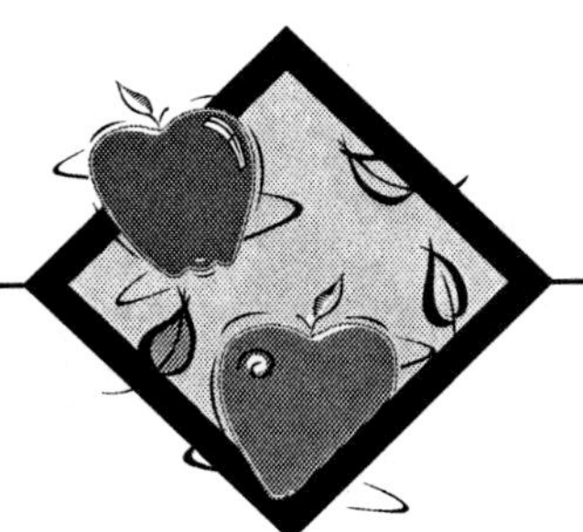

A Complete, Yet Simple, Book for Anyone Interested In Eating for Optimal Health; Includes Eating for Fitness and Sport

Cherie L. Moore
Cuesta College

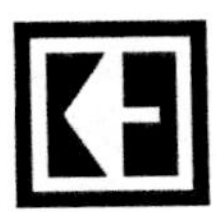

KENDALL/HUNT PUBLISHING COMPANY
4050 Westmark Drive Dubuque, Iowa 52002

ISBN: 978-0-7575-3754-7

Printed in the United States of America
10 9 8 7

Contents

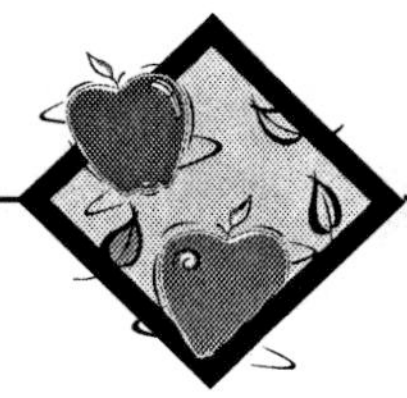

Foreword

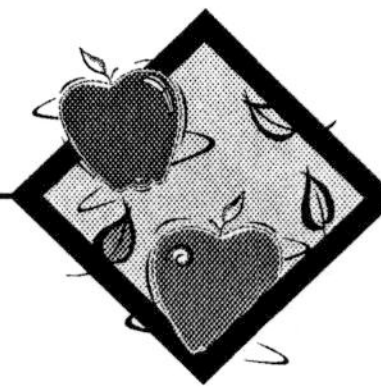

Increasingly people are coming to realize that diet, exercise, and attitude have everything to do with lasting good health. With the pace that most people keep in managing their lives, it is difficult to know where to start improving their diets. Fat loss, disease prevention, and improved sports performance are not gained from food restriction, but can be achieved by choosing healthful foods that can be eaten in abundance. *Practical Nutrition for a Fit Life* is a complete, yet simple, book for anyone interested in eating for optimal health and includes eating for fitness and sport. In a time when people mistakenly believe that carbohydrates are bad, it is refreshing to have a book that focuses on nutritional truths and applicable information. This is the first nutrition book that takes you step-by-step through nutritional information, and then how to evaluate your diet with a software program and set goals for change. It allows you to calculate your nutritional needs and personalize a diet that fits your needs.

Although the book is being used in both General Nutrition and Sports Nutrition college classes, anyone will benefit. The Personal Assessment tear-out sheets in chapter 19 have been included for classroom purposes or for you to use on your own. The final chapter is a template for a diet analysis of your own personal diet so that you may apply the information learned on your road to fitness!

About the Author

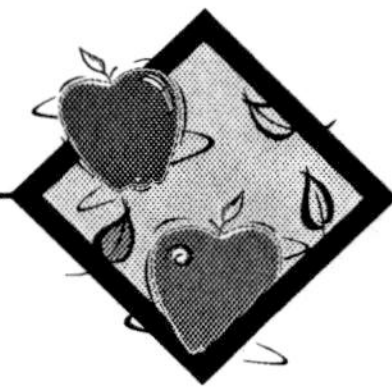

Cherie Moore received her bachelor's degree in Exercise Physiology and Nutrition from the University of Hawaii in 1985. She received a Teaching Credential in Nutrition, Health, and Physical Education from Chapman College in Orange, California, in 1990. She completed her master's degree in Wellness Management (with a thesis developing an ultramarathon food replacement drink) from Cal Poly, San Luis Obispo, California, in 1992. Cherie has been working in the fitness and nutrition field since 1981 as a certified fitness instructor, nutrition consultant, aerobic director, fitness studio owner, ESPN Bodies in Motion demonstrator, weight-training supervisor, head track and field coach, dance instructor, nutrition guest speaker, elementary PE teacher, certified soccer coach, high school health teacher, nutrition instructor, and developed some of the original aerobic and personal training certification exams and first stationary bicycle interval/music workouts in 1991. Cherie also completed the Center for Lactation Education Lactation Consultant coursework and has been teaching nutrition full time at Cuesta College in California since 1992. Two of Cherie's nutrition specialty areas are sports nutrition and maternal and child nutrition, which have inspired her to develop these classes at Cuesta College and may be taken online from anywhere in the world.

Cherie enjoys cycling, swimming, running, weight training, kayaking, hiking, camping, and triathlons, and she has competed in numerous ultramarathon cycling events. Her most notable cycling accomplishments include setting a transcontinental tandem cycling record in 1986 with another female and winning the tandem division of the Race Across America with her husband in 1991. Combining her education background with her personal experiences Cherie is able to convey nutritional information for both athletes and active people in an easy-to-read practical format.

chapter 1

Connecting Health and Nutrition—The Big Picture

The Link Between Health and Nutrition

To study nutrition, you may first want to consider the bigger picture of how nutrition fits into your overall health. As you learn about health and nutrition, you will see how they are connected. Inadequate or improper nutrition is associated with the three leading causes of death and disease in our country (heart disease, cancer, and stroke), which are largely associated with our lifestyle choices.

Actually, all of the 10 leading causes of death in our country can be related to lifestyle practices. Heart disease, cancer, stroke, chronic obstructive lung disease, unintentional injuries, pneumonia and influenza, diabetes mellitus, HIV infection, suicide, and homicide can be linked to either dietary choices, lack of activity, alcohol intake, drug consumption, or smoking. The causes of death and the diseases related to improper diet and/or lack of physical activity are appear in the box that follows.

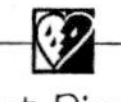

Heart Disease
Cancer
Stroke
Hypertension
Diabetes
Obesity
Arthritis
Osteoporosis

It has been estimated that these chronic diseases cause over 80% of all deaths in our country and that 60% to 90% of all deaths are likely caused by lifestyle (everyday) habits, especially nutritional habits. For example, richer societies tend to eat more fat and more animal products, which results in more bowel disease as well as medical conditions and many types of cancer. However, with the epidemic spread of cheap high-fat fast food in foreign countries, they too are able to suffer from these diseases. Prevention strategies within our lifestyle habits are the best approach for lessening our chances of developing these diseases. Physical activity and diet are two of the leading lifestyle factors in preventing chronic disease and death in our country.

What Is Health and Nutrition?

The World Health Organization states that *"health is not merely the absence of disease, but the state of complete mental, social, and physical well-being."* To achieve optimal health, you might strive to achieve increased thinking abilities, increased physical fitness, increased coping abilities, increased social fitness, increased spiritual fitness, increased energy levels, as well as the decreased risk of disease.

The Council on Food and Nutrition of the American Medical Association states nutrition as meaning *"the science of food, the nutrients and the substances therein, their action, interaction, and balance in relation to health and disease, and the process by which the organism ingests, absorbs, transports, utilizes, and excretes food substances."*

Each nutrient has specific functions in the body that contribute to these optimal health goals. The imbalance of the nutrients also contributes to many types of diseases. Too much of a nutrient sometimes can cause as many problems as not enough. This book will help you understand the foods to eat to obtain the desired balance of nutrients for optimal health.

Two researchers have made comments related to the great impact of lifestyle changes on your health and specifically your chance of having illness and death. Donald Ardell says, "People don't die, they kill themselves—the most lethal illnesses are the diseases of choice, related to our lifestyle" and a researcher, Knowles states, "Over 99% of us are born healthy and made sick as a result of misbehavior and environmental conditions." These are both profound statements that reflect the role we play in our own health. It is largely up to us whether we develop heart disease, diabetes, obesity, or colon cancer. Now that you are ready to make the most healthful choices for optimal health, how do you know what those food choices should be?

Learning about Health, Fitness, and Nutrition

To learn about what causes disease and how nutrition links to health, scientists use the scientific method while doing research and report their findings in peer-reviewed journals. The nutrition field, especially sports nutrition, is full of "quackery" products in which a company is making unproven claims on a product to entice a person to buy it, when it is likely that the product is useless.

Scientific research studies are continually submitted and reflect the current state of nutrition knowledge available. Laboratory studies are common when attempting to find out what nutritional substances may cause cancer in rats and therefore possibly also cause cancer in humans. Case studies are done for individual situations, but may not be of value unless several case studies can be compared. Epidemiological studies use certain populations to determine the relationship of various risk factors to diseases or health problems. An example would be comparing the U.S. diet to the diet of southern Italy and finding that people in the United States have a much higher heart disease rate and a much higher saturated fat intake. Intervention or experimental studies manipulate an independent variable to observe the outcome in a dependent variable. This would be to discover a cause-and-effect relationship. When done blindly (without the subjects of the study knowing their role or product in the study), then results of well-controlled experimental studies can be considered valid.

The **Scientific Method** involves the following steps:

- **A Question is asked**
- **A Hypothesis is generated**
- **Research is conducted**
- **Conclusions are made**
- **Findings are Peer evaluated**
- **Follow-up Experiments are completed.**

Consumers are bombarded by supplement companies, advertisements, and sometimes coaching recommendations to try a particular product. Nutritional quackery is especially rampant in the sports nutrition field because top athletes who are similar in genetics and equipment are looking for the competitive edge, and supplement manufacturers want to profit from this attitude.

Some elements of **nutritional quackery** are the following:

- **The claim is too good to be true.**
- **It claims to have a secret formula.**
- **It makes unrealistic guarantees.**
- **It claims weight loss > a pound a week.**
- **It uses "star" testimonials.**
- **It claims that nonessential nutrients are essential.**

Sometimes evaluating claims can be difficult because it is not easy to control all the variables in studies with human beings; numerous physiological, psychological, and biomechanical factors influence athletic performance and vary from day to day; and the results of one study with humans does not prove anything. Remember, "Buyer beware."

Learning What to Eat

For you to go about learning what and how much to eat, you would first need to learn the body's nutrient needs, then categorize those needs, then learn the foods to meet those needs. Additionally if you learn how to think critically about food choices, read labels, and evaluate foods, then you are ready to apply all this information to create your own personalized food plan.

The Body's Nutrient Needs

About 45 essential nutrients need to be obtained either from the diet or supplements. Those nutrients include glucose, 2 essential fatty acids, 9 essential amino acids, 13 vitamins, about 21 minerals, and water. The simple classification categories for these nutrients are the following:

- **Carbohydrates**
- **Fats (lipids)**
- **Protein**
- **Vitamins**
- **Minerals**
- **Water**

All of these are essential for every cell in the body and for human life to exist. Three of them contain calories.

What Is a Calorie and Which Nutrients Contain Calories?

A Calorie in nutrition is a measurement of energy measured in a bomb calorimeter that measures the amount of heat it takes to raise the temperature of 1 gram of water by 1 degree Celsius. Food is measured in **kilocalories (kcal)**. "Calories" with a large "C" on nutrition label are the same as kilocalories.

The three nutrients that are classified as energy nutrients and provide Calories to fuel the cells are carbohydrates, lipids, and proteins. Carbohydrates provide 4 Calories per gram and can be generally classified as "complex" or "simple," which will be explained in detail in chapter 4. Active people and athletes should consume a majority (65%–75%) of their Calories from carbohydrates. Lipids provide 9 Calories per gram and can be generally classified as unsaturated or saturated when discussing the fatty acid makeup of triglycerides. The government recommends less that 30% of Calories come from lipids, but many nutritionists recommend less than 20%. Proteins offer 4 Calories per gram and will be approximately 10%–15% of one's Calories if the appropriate grams for the amount of Calories are chosen. A fourth contributor to energy is a toxin called alcohol that provides 7 Calories per gram, but is not considered a nutrient. The nutritive caloric components will be discussed in detail in following chapters.

The Standard American Diet (SAD Diet) energy nutrient breakdown is quite different than the recommendations given. It is composed primarily of animal fats, animal protein, and simple and refined carbohydrates. Vegetables, fruits, and whole grains are rarely consumed in an adequate quantity in the average American's diet (the term *American* is referring to just the United States).

Energy Nutrient Calculations

In order to calculate the percentage of Calories of each energy nutrient in a product or in one's diet, one can use the 4/4/9 Calories per gram conversions to calculate the Calories of a product or a day's food diary. For example, you may eat 290 grams of carbohydrates, 60 grams of fat, and 70 grams of protein in one day. The first step is to find the Calories for each of the energy-yielding nutrients:

CHO	290 grams × 4 kcal/g	= 1160 kcal
Fat	60 grams × 9 kcal/g	= 540 kcal
Protein	70 grams × 4 kcal/g	= 280 kcal

Then total the Calories:

Total	1980 kcal

You can then calculate the percentage of fats, carbohydrates, and proteins by doing a basic percentage problem dividing each of the Calories separately by the total Calories.

% kcal from CHO	=	1160/1980	=	59% of Calories from carbs
% kcal from fat	=	540/1980	=	27% of Calories from fat
% kcal from protein	=	280/1980	=	14% of Calories from protein

Non-Energy-Yielding Nutrients

Organic **fat and water-soluble vitamins** and inorganic **trace and major minerals** do not provide energy in Calories, but they are vital in the body's metabolic functioning. Water is the sixth category of nutrient and vital to the life of every cell in the body. It is a solvent, lubricant, medium for transport, and temperature regulator that makes up the majority (about two-thirds) of our body and yields no energy. Therefore, the nutrients in foods offer not only energy for every cell in the body, but also the growth and repair of tissue, the regulating of metabolism, and to provide water for every cell. The specific details of vitamins and minerals and fluid balance will be explained in later chapters as well.

Making Food Choices

Many factors influence our food choices such as childhood experiences, peer influences, education, income amount, health reasons, and the convenience factor. In the attempt to avoid the leading causes of death in our country, you might learn to recognize these influences and combine them with the practice of healthful nutrition habits and the goal of healthful nutrition and wellness for a fit life.

chapter 2

Tools for Designing Diets

Health and Nutrition Assessment

Several tools can be used to evaluate and design diets. Before learning and using these tools, the status of your health may be assessed as "desirable," "undernutrition," or "overnutrition." The condition of undernutrition may lead to depleted nutrient stores and reduced biochemical functions that become measurable by clinical signs and symptoms. The condition of overnutrition may be caused by excess Calories and fat and lead to obesity. It may also involve excessive use of vitamins and minerals that leads to imbalances or toxicities, although excess energy is the most common condition in the United States.

One's nutritional status can be assessed by the **ABCDE method**. **Anthropometrics** includes measurements such as weight and height. A **biochemical** analysis includes blood and urine tests. Doctors, specifically Endocrinologists, will assess your blood work. **Clinical** assessment includes recognizing signs and symptoms of deficiencies or excesses. Many NDs (Naturopathic Doctors) will use clinical assessment techniques to assess health status. **Diet** history, often used by a dietician or nutritionist, is a method of assessment that looks at what a person has been eating that when combined with other methods of assessment, helps in evaluating the overall picture of assessment. **Economic** status is an additional factor when assessing your nutritional intake since malnutrition occurs more frequently in lower income families.

When looking at the current status of the health of Americans in the United States, studies show a small improvement in the reduction of fat and cholesterol in their diets, but obesity has become an epidemic; more people are sedentary (computers and TV contributing greatly), few people eat a minimal of five vegetables and fruits daily, and few people eat whole grains.

Nutrient Recommendations

As stated in Chapter 1, in order to learn what and how much to eat, you would first learn the body's nutrient needs, and next categorize those needs, then learn the foods to meet those needs. Additionally, if you learn how to think critically about food choices, read labels, and evaluate foods, then you are ready to apply all of this information to create a personalized food plan.

The Food and Nutrition Board of the National Academy of Sciences unites with the United States Department of Agriculture and many other organizations to study and establish guidelines (originally Recommended Dietary Allowances; now the overall umbrella term for recommendations is called the **DRIs for Dietary Reference Intakes**) for each nutrient that is essential (vital for life and not made by the body). These guidelines meet the general nutrition needs of healthy adults. Many people have criticized the RDA's, but the Food and Nutrition Board has separated the nutrients that they still need more research on and give an estimated safe and **Adequate Intake (AI)** for those. The Food and Nutrition Board has also established **Tolerable Upper Intake Levels (UL)** for those nutrients that are known to be toxic at certain levels. The following charts give the current DRI's established by the Food and Nutrition Board:

Dietary Reference Intakes (DRIs): Recommended Intakes for Individuals, Elements

Food and Nutrition Board, Institute of Medicine, National Academies

Life Stage Group	Calcium (mg/d)	Chromium (μg/d)	Copper (μg/d)	Fluoride (mg/d)	Iodine (μg/d)	Iron (mg/d)	Magnesium (mg/d)	Manganese (mg/d)	Molybdenum (μg/d)	Phosphorus (mg/d)	Selenium (μg/d)	Zinc (mg/d)
Infants												
0–6 mo	210*	0.2*	200*	0.01*	110*	0.27*	30*	0.003*	2*	100*	15*	2*
7–12 mo	270*	5.5*	220*	0.5*	130*	**11**	75*	0.6*	3*	275*	20*	**3**
Children												
1–3 y	500*	11*	**340**	0.7*	**90**	**7**	**80**	1.2*	**17**	**460**	**20**	**3**
4–8 y	800*	15*	**440**	1*	**90**	**10**	**130**	1.5*	**22**	**500**	**30**	**5**
Males												
9–13 y	1,300*	25*	**700**	2*	**120**	**8**	**240**	1.9*	**34**	**1,250**	**40**	**8**
4–18 y	1,300*	35*	**890**	3*	**150**	**11**	**410**	2.2*	**43**	**1,250**	**55**	**11**
19–30 y	1,000*	35*	**900**	4*	**150**	**8**	**400**	2.3*	**45**	**700**	**55**	**11**
31–50 y	1,000*	35*	**900**	4*	**150**	**8**	**420**	2.3*	**45**	**700**	**55**	**11**
51–70 y	1,200*	30*	**900**	4*	**150**	**8**	**420**	2.3*	**45**	**700**	**55**	**11**
> 70 y	1,200*	30*	**900**	4*	**150**	**8**	**420**	2.3*	**45**	**700**	**55**	**11**
Females												
9–13 y	1,300*	21*	**700**	2*	**120**	**8**	**240**	1.6*	**34**	**1,250**	**40**	**8**
14–18 y	1,300*	24*	**890**	3*	**150**	**15**	**360**	1.6*	**43**	**1,250**	**55**	**9**
19–30 y	1,000*	25*	**900**	3*	**150**	**18**	**310**	1.8*	**45**	**700**	**55**	**8**
31–50 y	1,000*	25*	**900**	3*	**150**	**18**	**320**	1.8*	**45**	**700**	**55**	**8**
51–70 y	1,200*	20*	**900**	3*	**150**	**8**	**320**	1.8*	**45**	**700**	**55**	**8**
> 70 y	1,200*	20*	**900**	3*	**150**	**8**	**320**	1.8*	**45**	**700**	**55**	**8**
Pregnancy												
≤ 18 y	1,300*	29*	**1,000**	3*	**220**	**27**	**400**	2.0*	**50**	**1,250**	**60**	**12**
19–30 y	1,000*	30*	**1,000**	3*	**220**	**27**	**350**	2.0*	**50**	**700**	**60**	**11**
31–50 y	1,000*	30*	**1,000**	3*	**220**	**27**	**360**	2.0*	**50**	**700**	**60**	**11**
Lactation												
≤ 18 y	1,300*	44*	**1,300**	3*	**290**	**10**	**360**	2.6*	**50**	**1,250**	**70**	**13**
19–30 y	1,000*	45*	**1,300**	3*	**290**	**9**	**310**	2.6*	**50**	**700**	**70**	**12**
31–50 y	1,000*	45*	**1,300**	3*	**290**	**9**	**320**	2.6*	**50**	**700**	**70**	**12**

NOTE: This table presents Recommended Dietary Allowances (RDAs) in **bold type** and Adequate Intakes (AIs) in ordinary type followed by an asterisk (*). RDAs and AIs may both be used as goals for individual intake. RDAs are set to meet the needs of almost all (97 to 98 percent) individuals in a group. For healthy breastfed infants, the AI is the mean intake. The AI for other life stage and gender groups is believed to cover needs of all individuals in the group, but lack of data or uncertainty in the data prevent being able to specify with confidence the percentage of individuals covered by this intake.

SOURCES: Dietary Reference Intakes for Calcium, Phosphorus, Magnesium, Vitamin D, and Fluoride (1997); Dietary Reference Intakes for Thiamin, Riboflavin, Niacin, Vitamin B6, Folate, Vitamin B12, Pantothenic Acid, Biotin, and Choline (1998); Dietary Reference Intakes for Vitamin C, Vitamin E, Selenium, and Carotenoids (2000); and Dietary Reference Intakes for Vitamin A, Vitamin K, Arsenic, Boron, Chromium, Copper, Iodine, Iron, Manganese, Molybdenum, Nickel, Silicon, Vanadium, and Zinc (2001). These reports may be accessed via www.nap.edu.

Dietary Reference Intakes (DRIs): Recommended Intakes for Individuals, Vitamins

Food and Nutrition Board, Institute of Medicine, National Academies

Life Stage Group	Vitamin A (μg/d)[a]	Vitamin C (mg/d)	Vitamin D (μg/d)[b, c]	Vitamin E (mg/d)[d]	Vitamin K (μg/d)	Thiamin (mg/d)	Riboflavin (mg/d)	Niacin (mg/d)[e]	Vitamin B_6 (mg/d)	Folate (μg/d)[f]	Vitamin B_{12} (μg/d)	Pantothenic Acid (mg/d)	Biotin (μg/d)	Choline (mg/d)[g]
Infants														
0–6 mo	400*	40*	5*	4*	2.0*	0.2*	0.3*	2*	0.1*	65*	0.4*	1.7*	5*	125*
7–12 mo	500*	50*	5*	5*	2.5*	0.3*	0.4*	4*	0.3*	80*	0.5*	1.8*	6*	150*
Children														
1–3 y	300	15	5*	6	30*	0.5	0.5	6	0.5	150	0.9	2*	8*	200*
4–8 y	400	25	5*	7	55*	0.6	0.6	8	0.6	200	1.2	3*	12*	250*
Males														
9–13 y	600	45	5*	11	60*	0.9	0.9	12	1.0	300	1.8	4*	20*	375*
14–18 y	900	75	5*	15	75*	1.2	1.3	16	1.3	400	2.4	5*	25*	550*
19–30 y	900	90	5*	15	120*	1.2	1.3	16	1.3	400	2.4	5*	30*	550*
31–50 y	900	90	5*	15	120*	1.2	1.3	16	1.3	400	2.4	5*	30*	550*
51–70 y	900	90	10*	15	120*	1.2	1.3	16	1.7	400	2.4[h]	5*	30*	550*
> 70 y	900	90	15*	15	120*	1.2	1.3	16	1.7	400	2.4[h]	5*	30*	550*
Females														
9–13 y	600	45	5*	11	60*	0.9	0.9	12	1.0	300	1.8	4*	20*	375*
14–18 y	700	65	5*	15	75*	1.0	1.0	14	1.2	400[i]	2.4	5*	25*	400*
19–30 y	700	75	5*	15	90*	1.1	1.1	14	1.3	400[i]	2.4	5*	30*	425*
31–50 y	700	75	5*	15	90*	1.1	1.1	14	1.3	400[i]	2.4	5*	30*	425*
51–70 y	700	75	10*	15	90*	1.1	1.1	14	1.5	400	2.4[h]	5*	30*	425*
> 70 y	700	75	15*	15	90*	1.1	1.1	14	1.5	400	2.4[h]	5*	30*	425*
Pregnancy														
≤ 18 y	750	80	5*	15	75*	1.4	1.4	18	1.9	600[j]	2.6	6*	30*	450*
19–30 y	770	85	5*	15	90*	1.4	1.4	18	1.9	600[j]	2.6	6*	30*	450*
31–50 y	770	85	5*	15	90*	1.4	1.4	18	1.9	600[j]	2.6	6*	30*	450*
Lactation														
≤ 18 y	1,200	115	5*	19	75*	1.4	1.6	17	2.0	500	2.8	7*	35*	550*
19–30 y	1,300	120	5*	19	90*	1.4	1.6	17	2.0	500	2.8	7*	35*	550*
31–50 y	1,300	120	5*	19	90*	1.4	1.6	17	2.0	500	2.8	7*	35*	550*

mg = milligram, μg = microgram

NOTE: This table (taken from the DRI reports, see www.nap.edu) presents Recommended Dietary Allowances (RDAs) in **bold type** and Adequate Intakes (AIs) in ordinary type followed by an asterisk (*). RDAs and AIs may both be used as goals for individual intake. RDAs are set to meet the needs of almost all (97 to 98 percent) individuals in a group. For healthy breastfed infants, the AI is the mean intake. The AI for other life stage and gender groups is believed to cover needs of all individuals in the group, but lack of data or uncertainty in the data prevent being able to specify with confidence the percentage of individuals covered by this intake.

[a] As retinol activity equivalents (RAEs). 1 RAE = 1 μg retinol, 12 μg β-carotene, 24 μg α-carotene, or 24 μg β-cryptoxanthin. To calculate RAEs from REs of provitamin A carotenoids in foods, divide the REs by 2. For preformed vitamin A in foods or supplements and for provitamin A carotenoids in supplements, 1 RE = 1 RAE.

[b] cholecalciferol. 1 μg cholecalciferol = 40 IU vitamin D.

[c] In the absence of adequate exposure to sunlight.

[d] As α-tocopherol. α-Tocopherol includes *RRR*-α-tocopherol, the only form of α-tocopherol that occurs naturally in foods, and the *2R* stereoisomeric forms of α-tocopherol (*RRR*-, *RSR*-, *RRS*-, and *RSS*-α-tocopherol) that occur in fortified foods and supplements. It does not include the *2S*-stereoisomeric forms of α-tocopherol (*SRR*-, *SSR*-, *SRS*-, and *SSS*-α-tocopherol), also found in fortified foods and supplements.

[e] As niacin equivalents (NE). 1 mg of niacin = 60 mg of tryptophan; 0–6 months = preformed niacin (not NE).

[f] As dietary folate equivalents (DFE), 1 DFE = 1 μg food folate = 0.6 μg of folic acid from fortified food or as a supplement consumed with food = 0.5 μg of a supplement taken on an empty stomach.

[g] Although AIs have been set for choline, there are few data to assess whether a dietary supply of choline is needed at all stages of the life cycle, and it may be that the choline requirement can be met by endogenous synthesis at some of these stages.

[h] Because 10 to 30 percent of older people may malabsorb food-bound B_{12}, it is advisable far those older than 50 years to meet their RDA mainly by consuming foods fortified with B_{12} or a supplement containing B_{12}.

[i] In view of evidence linking folate intake with neural tube defects in the fetus, it is recommended that all women capable of becoming pregnant consume 400 μg from supplements or fortified foods in addition to intake of food folate from a varied diet.

[j] It is assumed that women will continue consuming 400 μg from supplements or fortified food until their pregnancy is confirmed and they enter prenatal care, which ordinarily occurs after the end of the periconceptional period—the critical time for formation of the neural tube.

Dietary Reference Intakes (DRIs): Tolerable Upper Intake Levels (UL[a]), Elements

Food and Nutrition Board, Institute of Medicine, National Academies

Life Stage Group	Arsenic[b]	Boron (mg/d)	Calcium (g/d)	Chromium	Copper (μg/d)	Fluoride (mg/d)	Iodine (μg/d)	Iron (mg/d)	Magnesium (mg/d)[c]	Manganese (mg/d)	Molybdenum (μg/d)	Nickel (mg/d)	Phosphorus (g/d)	Selenium (μg/d)	Silicon[d]	Vanadium (mg/d)[e]	Zinc (mg/d)
Infants																	
0–6 mo	ND	ND	ND	ND	ND	0.7	ND	40	ND	ND	ND	ND	ND	45	ND	ND	4
7–12 mo	ND	ND	ND	ND	ND	0.9	ND	40	ND	ND	ND	ND	ND	60	ND	ND	5
Children																	
1–3 y	ND	3	2.5	ND	1,000	1.3	200	40	65	2	300	0.2	3	90	ND	ND	7
4–8 y	ND	6	2.5	ND	3,000	2.2	300	40	110	3	600	0.3	3	150	ND	ND	12
Males, Females																	
9–13 y	ND	11	2.5	ND	5,000	10	600	40	350	6	1,100	0.6	4	280	ND	ND	23
14–18 y	ND	17	2.5	ND	8,000	10	900	45	350	9	1,700	1.0	4	400	ND	ND	34
19–70 y	ND	20	2.5	ND	10,000	10	1,100	45	350	11	2,000	1.0	4	400	ND	1.8	40
< 70 y	ND	20	2.5	ND	10,000	10	1,100	45	350	11	2,000	1.0	3	400	ND	1,8	40
Pregnancy																	
≤ 18 y	ND	17	2.5	ND	8,000	10	900	45	350	9	1,700	1.0	3.5	400	ND	ND	34
19–50 y	ND	20	2.5	ND	10,000	10	1,100	45	350	11	2,000	1.0	3.5	400	ND	ND	40
Lactation																	
≤ 18 y	ND	17	2.5	ND	8,000	10	900	45	350	9	1,700	1.0	4	400	ND	ND	34
19–50 y	ND	20	2.5	ND	10,000	10	1,100	45	350	11	2,000	1.0	4	400	ND	ND	40

[a]UL = The maximum level of daily nutrient intake that is likely to pose no risk of adverse effects. Unless otherwise specified, the UL represents total intake from food, water, and supplements. Due to lack of suitable data, ULs could not be established for arsenic, chromium, and silicon. In the absence of ULs, extra caution may be warranted in consuming levels above recommended intakes.

[b]Although the UL was not determined for arsenic, there is no justification for adding arsenic to food or supplements.

[c]The ULs for magnesium represent intake from a pharmacological agent only and do not include intake from food and water.

[d]Although silicon has not been shown to cause adverse effects in humans, there is no justification for adding silicon to supplements.

[e]Although vanadium in food has not been shown to cause adverse effects in humans, there is no justification for adding vanadium to food and vanadium supplements should be used with caution. The UL is based on adverse effects in laboratory animals and this data could be used to set a UL for adults but not children and adolescents.

[f]ND = Not determinable due to lack of data of adverse effects in this age group and concern with regard to lack of ability to handle excess amounts. Source of intake should be from food only to prevent high levels of intake.

SOURCES: Dietary Reference Intakes for Calcium, Phosphorus, Magnesium, Vitamin D, and Fluoride (1997); Dietary Reference Intakes for Thiamin, Riboflavin, Niacin, Vitamin B_6, Folate, Vitamin B_{12}, Pantothenic Acid, Biotin, and Choline (1998); Dietary Reference Intakes for Vitamin C, Vitamin E, Selenium, and Carotenoids (2000); and Dietary Reference Intakes for Vitamin A, Vitamin K, Arsenic, Boron, Chromium, Copper, Iodine, Iron, Manganese, Molybdenum, Nickel, Silicon, Vanadium, and Zinc (2001). These reports may be accessed via www.nap.edu.

Dietary Reference Intakes (DRIs): Tolerable Upper Intake Levels (UL[a]), Vitamins

Food and Nutrition Board, Institute of Medicine, National Academies

Life Stage Group	Vitamin A (μg/d)[b]	Vitamin C (mg/d)	Vitamin D (μg/d)	Vitamin E (mg/d)[c,d]	Vitamin K	Thiamin	Riboflavin	Niacin (mg/d)[d]	Vitamin B_6 (mg/d)	Folate (μg/d)[d]	Vitamin B_{12}	Pantothenic Acid	Biotin	Choline (g/d)	Carotenoids[e]
Infants															
0–6 mo	600	ND[f]	25	ND	ND	ND	ND	ND	ND	ND	ND	ND	ND	ND	ND
7–12 mo	600	ND	25	ND	ND	ND	ND	ND	ND	ND	ND	ND	ND	ND	ND
Children															
1–3 y	600	400	50	200	ND	ND	ND	10	30	300	ND	ND	ND	1.0	ND
4–8 y	900	650	50	300	ND	ND	ND	15	40	400	ND	ND	ND	1.0	ND
Males, Females															
9–13 y	1,700	1,200	50	600	ND	ND	ND	20	60	600	ND	ND	ND	2.0	ND
14–18 y	2,800	1,800	50	800	ND	ND	ND	30	80	800	ND	ND	ND	3.0	ND
19–70 y	3,000	2,000	50	1,000	ND	ND	ND	35	100	1,000	ND	ND	ND	3.5	ND
> 70 y	3,000	2,000	50	1,000	ND	ND	ND	35	100	1,000	ND	ND	ND	3.5	ND
Pregnancy															
≤ 18 y	2,800	1,800	50	800	ND	ND	ND	30	80	800	ND	ND	ND	3.0	ND
19–50 y	3,000	2,000	50	1,000	ND	ND	ND	35	100	1,000	ND	ND	ND	3.5	ND
Pregnancy															
≤ 18 y	2,800	1,800	50	800	ND	ND	ND	30	80	800	ND	ND	ND	3.0	ND
19–50 y	3,000	2,000	50	1,000	ND	ND	ND	35	100	1,000	ND	ND	ND	3.5	ND

[a]UL = The maximum level of daily nutrient intake that is likely to pose no risk of adverse effects. Unless otherwise specified, the UL represents total intake from food, water, and supplements. Due to lack of suitable data, ULs could not be established for vitamin K, thiamin, riboflavin, vitamin B_{12}, pantothenic acid, biotin, or carotenoids, In the absence of ULs, extra caution may be warranted in consuming levels above recommended intakes.

[b]As preformed vitamin A only.

[c]As α-tocopherol; applies to any form of supplemental α-tocopherol.

[d]The ULs for vitamin E, niacin, and folate apply to synthetic forms obtained from supplements, fortified foods, or a combination of the two.

[e]β-Carotene supplements are advised only to serve as a provitamin A source for individuals at risk of vitamin A deficiency.

[f]ND = Not determinable due to lack of data of adverse effects in this age group and concern with regard to lack of ability to handle excess amounts. Source of intake should be from food only to prevent high levels of intake.

SOURCES: Dietary Reference Intakes for Calcium, Phosphorus, Magnesium, Vitamin D, and Fluoride (1997); Dietary Reference Intakes for Thiamin, Riboflavin, Niacin, Vitamin B_6, Folate, Vitamin B_{12}, Pantothenic Acid, Biotin, and Choline (1998); Dietary Reference Intakes for Vitamin C, Vitamin E, Selenium, and Carotenoids (2000); and Dietary Reference Intakes for Vitamin A, Vitamin K, Arsenic, Boron, Chromium, Copper, Iodine, Iron, Manganese, Molybdenum, Nickel, Silicon, Vanadium, and Zinc (2001). These reports may be accessed via www.nap.edu.

Median Heights and Weights and Recommended Energy Intake

		Weight		Height		Average energy allowance (kcal)[b]			
Category	**Age (years) or condition**	**(kg)**	**(lb)**	**(cm)**	**(in)**	**REE[a] (kcal/day)**	**Multiples of REE**	**Per kg**	**Per day[c]**
Infants	0.0–0.5	6	13	60	24	320		108	650
	0.5–1.0	9	20	71	28	500		98	850
Children	1–3	13	29	90	35	740		102	1,300
	4–6	20	44	112	44	950		90	1,800
	7–10	28	62	132	52	1,130		70	2,000
Males	11–14	45	99	157	62	1,440	1.70	55	2,500
	15–18	66	145	176	69	1,760	1.67	45	3,000
	19–24	72	160	177	70	1,780	1.67	40	2,900
	25–50	79	174	176	70	1,800	1.60	37	2,900
	51+	77	170	173	68	1,530	1.50	30	2,300
Females	11–14	46	101	157	62	1,310	1.67	47	2,200
	15–18	55	120	163	64	1,370	1.60	40	2,200
	19–24	58	128	164	65	1,350	1.60	38	2,200
	25–50	63	138	163	64	1,380	1.55	36	2,200
	51+	65	143	160	63	1,280	1.50	30	1,900
Pregnant	1st trimester								+ 0
	2nd trimester								+ 300
	3rd trimester								+ 300
Lactating	1st 6 months								+ 500
	2nd 6 months								+ 500

[a]REE is resting energy expenditure; see chapter 15 for explanation. Calculation is based on Food and Agriculture Organization equations, then rounded.

[b]In the range of light to moderate activity, the coefficient of variation is ± 20%. Thus, for an individual with an average energy allowance of 2,500 Calories per day, the typical range might be 2,000–3,000, which is plus or minus 500 Calories (.20 × 32,500). See chapter 15 for expanded discussion of energy requirement based upon physical activity levels.

[c]Figure is rounded.

Protein, carbohydrate, and many vitamin and mineral needs may be increased for active people, but these should be easily attainable through the increase in Calories that active people need. When you want to assess your diet for total daily nutrient intakes, it is recommended to average at least three days of your dietary intake to calculate daily nutrient intakes since food intakes vary from day to day.

The DRIs are not only used for personal assessment, but they are also used for planning food supplies for groups, establishing standards for food assistance programs, evaluating dietary survey data, developing food and nutrition information, helping establish food label standards, regulating food fortification, and developing new food products.

Although they are used for developing food products and helping to establish food label standards, the DRI's are not used on a food label because it is gender and age specific in the charts and it would require too many categories to fit on a label. Therefore, the FDA developed **Daily Values (DV)** for food labels that include **Reference Daily Intakes (RDI)** for vitamins and minerals and **Daily Reference Values (DRV)** for nutrients without DRIs such as those listed in the chart to the right.

Food Component	DRV 2000 kcal
Fat	< 65 g
Sat. Fat	< 20 g
Protein	50 g
Cholesterol	< 300 mg
CHO	300 g
Fiber	25 g
Sodium	< 2400 mg
Potassium	3500 mg

Detailed food label information will be given in Chapter 14, Consumer Nutrition.

Foods That Meet the Nutrient Needs

The next step in designing your diet is to choose the foods that will help meet your established nutrient needs. There are many planning tools or methods for designing a dietary plan. The **Nutrient Density Concept** involves simply choosing foods with a high nutrient density (a lot of nutrients proportionally to the amount of Calories). Examples of nutrient dense foods would be broccoli, carrots, and lentils. Another tool is to follow the **Dietary Guidelines**, which vary from source to source, but are generally similar with each other (excluding fad diets such as "No carb" types). Another tool is to utilize a visual **Food Guide** such as one of the pyramids or **The Healthful House of Food and Fitness**. **Food Exchange Lists** are another format that is more specific to caloric distribution than the food pyramids. Lastly, and probably a more accurate method for assessing and designing dietary plans are using **Computer Diet Analysis** programs to assess, evaluate, and make changes to match one's personal nutrient and caloric needs.

Dietary Guidelines

The Dietary Guidelines of 2000 were divided into three categories with several sub-categories. Under **Aim For Fitness** was "Aim for a healthy weight" and "Be physically active each day." To achieve this one would balance Calories in with Calories out and strive for exercising 30 minutes on most days, even if it is for 3x10-minute intervals of walking. Under the second part of the guidelines, **Build a Healthy Base**, was "Let the pyramids guide your food choices," "Choose a variety of grains daily, especially whole grains," "Choose a variety of fruits and veggies daily" and "Keep food safe to eat." Under the third part of the guidelines, **Choose Sensibly**, was "Choose a diet that is low in saturated fat and cholesterol and moderate in total fat," "Choose beverages and foods to moderate your intake of sugars," "Choose and prepare foods with less salt," "If you drink alcoholic beverages, do so in moderation (but not at all if you are pregnant)."

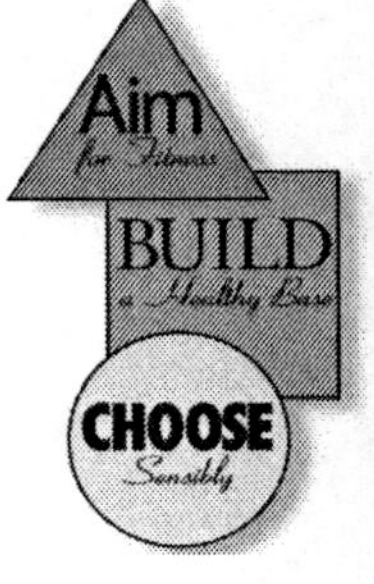

Logo for Dietary Guidelines

The Eatwise Dietary Guidelines, developed by the Oldways Preservation Trust and Exchange Organization, which make recommendations to the government for dietary guidelines and have developed the food pyramids based on other countries. The *Eatwise* Dietary Guidelines for People who enjoy Lifelong Good Health are:

- **They eat grains and related foods at each meal, mainly whole grain, unrefined, and minimally processed.**
- **They eat a variety of fruits and vegetables, about seven cups throughout the day.**
- **They eat mostly legumes, nuts and seeds, then fish, poultry, and then less often, red meat.**

- **They eat moderate amounts of fats, preferably plant oils over animal fats.**
- **They eat small amounts of dairy foods, mostly as yogurt and cheese and wise eaters know that soy milk are healthful alternatives.**
- **They eat small amounts of added sugar and added salt.**
- **They drink about six glasses of water a day, and if they drink alcohol, they do so in moderation (but none at all if pregnant).**
- **They enjoy their pleasures of their foods and meals.**
- **They emphasize breastfeeding as the best start in life.**
- **They support vegetarianism; emphasizing plant foods over animal foods.**
- **They encourage sustainability by buying local and sustainable foods.**
- **They encourage safe and hygienic foods by practicing food safety at home.**

The newest dietary guidelines of 2005 build upon the previous Eatwise and 2000 guidelines with the following key recommendations:

Dietary Guidelines for Americans 2005

Key Recommendations for the General Population

Adequate Nutrients within Calorie Needs

- Consume a variety of nutrient-dense foods and beverages within and among the basic food groups while choosing foods that limit the intake of saturated and *trans* fats, cholesterol, added sugars, salt, and alcohol.
- Meet recommended intakes within energy needs by adopting a balanced eating pattern, such as the U.S. Department of Agriculture (USDA) Food Guide or the Dietary Approaches to Stop Hypertension (DASH) Eating Plan.

Weight Management

- To maintain body weight in a healthy range, balance calories from foods and beverages with calories expended.
- To prevent gradual weight gain over time, make small decreases in food and beverage calories and increase physical activity.

Physical Activity

- Engage in regular physical activity and reduce sedentary activities to promote health, psychological well-being, and a healthy body weight.
  - To reduce the risk of chronic disease in adulthood: Engage in at least 30 minutes of moderate-intensity physical activity, above usual activity, at work or home on most days of the week.
  - For most people, greater health benefits can be obtained by engaging in physical activity of more vigorous intensity or longer duration.
  - To help manage body weight and prevent gradual, unhealthy body weight gain in adulthood: Engage in approximately 60 minutes of moderate- to vigorous-intensity activity on most days of the week while not exceeding caloric intake requirements.
  - To sustain weight loss in adulthood: Participate in at least 60 to 90 minutes of daily moderate-intensity physical activity while not exceeding caloric intake requirements. Some people may need to consult with a healthcare provider before participating in this level of activity.
- Achieve physical fitness by including cardiovascular conditioning, stretching exercises for flexibility, and resistance exercises or calisthenics for muscle strength and endurance.

Food Groups to Encourage

- Consume a sufficient amount of fruits and vegetables while staying within energy needs. Two cups of fruit and 2½ cups of vegetables per day are recommended for a reference 2,000-calorie intake, with higher or lower amounts depending on the calorie level.
- Choose a variety of fruits and vegetables each day. In particular, select from all five vegetable subgroups (dark green, orange, legumes, starchy vegetables, and other vegetables) several times a week.
- Consume 3 or more ounce-equivalents of whole-grain products per day, with the rest of the recommended grains coming from enriched or whole-grain products. In general, at least half the grains should come from whole grains.
- Consume 3 cups per day of fat-free or low-fat milk or equivalent milk products (or calcium-rich foods).

Fats

- Consume less than 10 percent of calories from saturated fatty acids and less than 300 mg/day of cholesterol, and keep *trans* fatty acid consumption as low as possible.
- Keep total fat intake between 20 to 35 percent of calories, with most fats coming from sources of polyunsaturated and monounsaturated fatty acids, such as fish, nuts, and vegetable oils.
- When selecting and preparing meat, poultry, dry beans, and milk or milk products, make choices that are lean, low-fat, or fat-free.
- Limit intake of fats and oils high in saturated and/or *trans* fatty acids, and choose products low in such fats and oils.

Carbohydrates

- Choose fiber-rich fruits, vegetables, and whole grains often.
- Choose and prepare foods and beverages with little added sugars or caloric sweeteners, such as amounts suggested by the USDA Food Guides and the DASH Eating Plan.
- Reduce the incidence of dental caries by practicing good oral hygiene and consuming sugar- and starch-containing foods and beverages less frequently.

Sodium and Potassium

- Consume less than 2,300 mg (approximately 1 teaspoon of salt) of sodium per day.
- Choose and prepare foods with little salt. At the same time, consume potassium-rich foods, such as fruits and vegetables.

Alcoholic Beverages

- Those who choose to drink alcoholic beverages should do so sensibly and in moderation—defined as the consumption of up to one drink per day for women and up to two drinks per day for men.
- Alcoholic beverages should not be consumed by some individuals, including those who cannot restrict their alcohol intake, women of childbearing age who may become pregnant, pregnant and lactating women, children and adolescents, individuals taking medications that can interact with alcohol, and those with specific medical conditions.
- Alcoholic beverages should be avoided by individuals engaging in activities that require attention, skill, or coordination, such as driving or operating machinery.

Food Safety

- To avoid microbial foodborne illness:
  - Clean hands, food contact surfaces, and fruits and vegetables. Meat and poultry should not be washed or rinsed.

- ◇ Separate raw, cooked, and ready-to-eat foods while shopping, preparing, or storing foods.
- ◇ Cook foods to a safe temperature to kill microorganisms.
- ◇ Chill (refrigerate) perishable food promptly and defrost foods properly.
- ◇ Avoid raw (unpasteurized) milk or any products made from unpasteurized milk, raw or partially cooked eggs or foods containing raw eggs, raw or undercooked meat and poultry, unpasteurized juices, and raw sprouts.

Note: The Dietary Guidelines for Americans 2005 *contains additional recommendations for specific populations. The full document is available at www.healthierus.gov/dietaryguidelines.*

Food Guides Galore

More detailed than the dietary guidelines is the practice of putting foods into a format so that people can easily visualize what foods they should eat. Categorizing foods into groups started in 1916 and continues today. The first government-suggested plan was the Five Group Plan that even included butter as a group; then there were seven (butter and sweets each had their own recommended group); next came the ever-popular Basic 4 that gave equal billing to the meat and milk groups as the grain, fruits, and vegetables. The Basic 4 has been blamed for the increase of heart disease and the obesity epidemic in our country. In 1992, the **USDA Food Pyramid** has replaced the **Basic 4**, although strong lobbying in Washington, DC by the Meat and Dairy representatives fought the change. In 2005, the **MyPyramid** replaced the USDA Food Guide Pyramid. Among the many food pyramids that were designed after the USDA pyramid was the Harvard School of Public Health **Latin American**, **Mediterranean**, **Asian**, and **Vegetarian pyramids** that are based on those diets around the world that follow the food choices in the pyramid and consequently have low disease rates. There is also the **Physician's Committee For Responsible Medicine's New Basic Four**, in which this national organization of about 5,000 medical doctors believe that legumes, whole grains, vegetables and fruits should be the four groups emphasized in your diet. The instructor, Cherie Moore, has designed the **Healthful House of Food and Fitness** that is more detailed than other food guides and caters more to health/nutrition-committed individuals or athletes wanting the optimal diet.

Athletes and active people could use any of these food guides to serve as a basic guide, but they would likely benefit most from the non-USDA pyramids that focus on more plant-based/high unrefined complex carbohydrate foods. However, healthful snack food examples in the old USDA guides could have included whole grain bagels, granola, and crackers at the base, melon, strawberries, carrots, peppers, and cherry tomatoes at the next level, then calcium-rich almond butter and vanilla soy yogurt as the calcium/dairy group, baked tofu and mashed pinto bean dip as the healthful proteins, and fresh guacamole (avocado) at the top for the healthful fat:

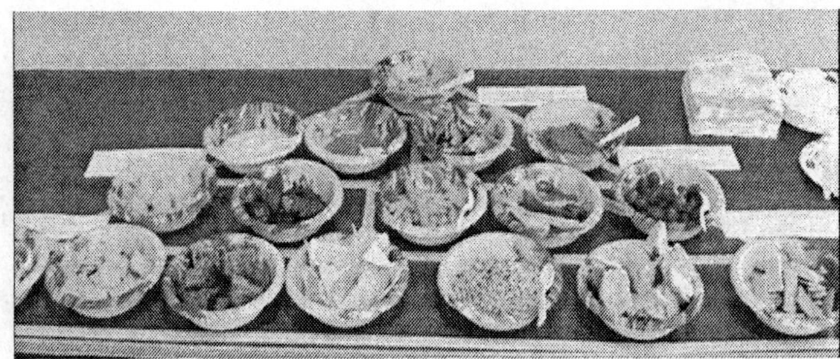

As the USDA food pyramid was designed to take the place of the old basic four plan, it also helped to translate science into more practical terms and to help people meet their nutritional needs for carbohydrate, protein, fat, vitamins, and minerals. The USDA Food Guide Pyramid was an improvement over the Old Basic Four food groups, but many nutritionists believed there was still work to be done. Most people did not make the choices given in the snack examples and did not realize that Americans were getting most of their fat from the meat and dairy—not the top of the pyramid.

Also, the "Meat" or "Protein" category combined beans, red meat, fish, and eggs in the same category whereas they are more different than they are alike. Beans and bean products are high fiber, low fat, low saturated fat, no cholesterol, and nutrient dense (contain many nutrients for the amount of Calories). Whereas red meat contains no fiber, and is high in total fat, saturated fat, and cholesterol. The USDA Pyramid also neglected to distinguish between different types of food in each category.

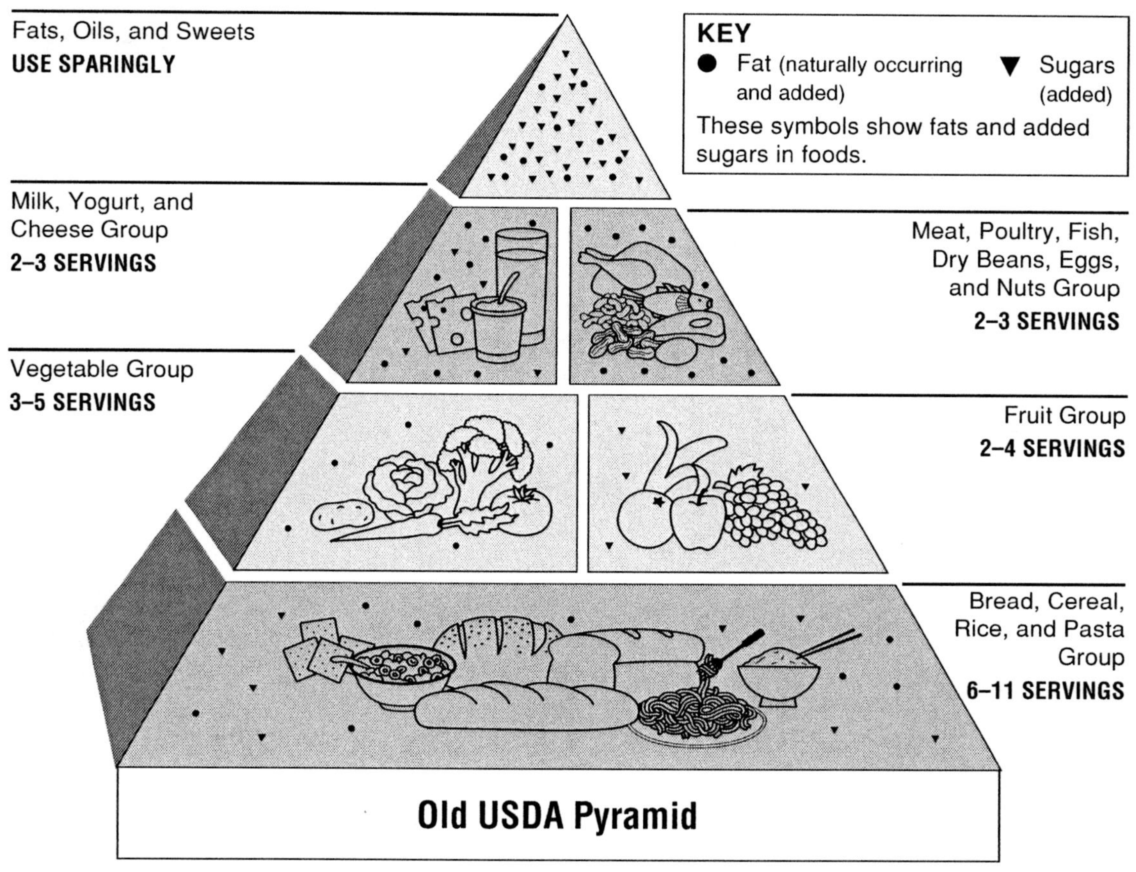

In addition to Calorie and nutrient variations within each group and the lack of specific guidelines for the most healthful choices in each group, this Pyramid was not (nor is the MyPyramid now) for children under the age of 2, who need almost half their Calories from fat (preferably healthful fats such as avocado, nut butters, olive oil and mother's milk). No one food contains every nutrient and variety within each group is important (such as a variety of all seven colors of fruits and vegetables for the full range of disease-fighting phytonutrients in the different colors). Americans never actually practiced the Food Guide Pyramid philosophy. They did not meet all the serving recommendations for all food groups; they consumed 1–2 servings of fruit a day (versus recommended 2–4), they consumed 2–3 servings of vegetables a day (versus recommended 3–5), and excessive intake in the fats, oils, and sweets group (versus use "sparingly") and excessive intake of high fat meats and refined grains. The old USDA Pyramid used the concept of "serving sizes" and what counted as a serving. Now in the MyPyramid, grains and proteins are measured in ounces, whereas fruits and vegetables and milk are measured in cups. The old USDA offered three caloric recommendation levels indicating the number of servings corresponding with one's caloric needs, and now offers 12 caloric levels with the new MyPyramid guidelines.

Anatomy of MyPyramid

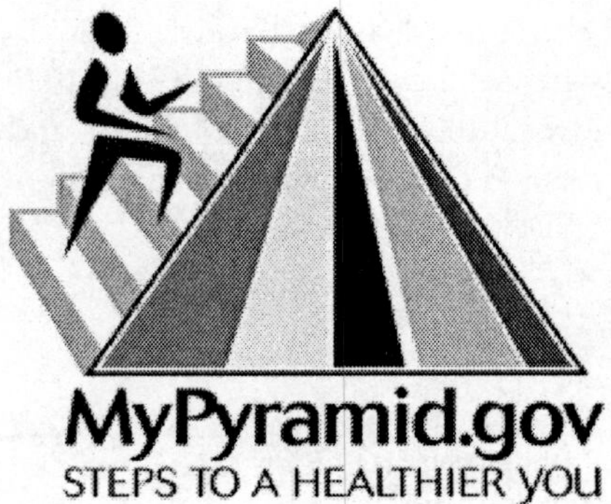

One Size Doesn't Fit All

USDA's new MyPyramid symbolizes a personalized approach to healthy eating and physical activity. The symbol has been designed to be simple. It has been developed to remind consumers to make healthful food choices and to be active every day. The different parts of the symbol are described below.

Activity

Activity is represented by the steps and the person climbing them, as a reminder of the importance of daily physical activity.

Moderation

Moderation is represented by the narrowing of each food group from bottom to top. The wider base stands for foods with little or no solid fats or added sugars. These should be selected more often. The narrower top area stands for foods containing more added sugars and solid fats. The more active you are, the more these foods can fit into your diet.

Personalization

Personalization is shown by the person on the steps, the slogan, and the URL. Find the kinds of amounts of food to eat each day at MyPyramid.gov.

Proportionality

Proportionality is shown by the different widths of the food group bands. The widths suggest how much food a person should choose from each group. The widths are just a general guide, not exact proportions. Check the Web site for how much is right for you.

Variety

Variety is symbolized by the six color bands representing the five food groups of the Pyramid and oils. This illustrates that foods from all groups are encouraged each day for good health.

Gradual Improvement

Gradual improvement is encouraged by the slogan. It suggests that individuals can benefit from taking small steps to improve their diet and lifestyle each day.

MyPyramid Food Intake Patterns

The suggested amounts of food to consume from the basic food groups, subgroups, and oils to meet recommended nutrient intakes are at 12 different calorie levels. Nutrient and energy contributions from each group are calculated according to the nutrient-dense forms of foods in each group (e.g., lean meats and fat-free milk). The table also shows the discretionary calorie allowance that can be accommodated within each calorie level, in addition to the suggested amounts of nutrient-dense forms of foods in each group.

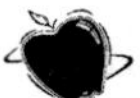

Daily Amount of Food From Each Group

Calorie Level[1]	1,000	1,200	1,400	1,600	1,800	2,000
Fruits[2]	1 cup	1 cup	1.5 cups	1.5 cups	1.5 cups	2 cups
Vegetables[3]	1 cup	1.5 cups	1.5 cups	2 cups	2.5 cups	2.5 cups
Grains[4]	3 oz–eq	4 oz–eq	5 oz–eq	5 oz–eq	6 oz–eq	6 oz–eq
Meat and Beans[5]	2 oz–eq	3 oz–eq	4 oz–eq	5 oz–eq	5 oz–eq	5.5 oz–eq
Milk[6]	2 cups	2 cups	2 cups	3 cups	3 cups	3 cups
Oils[7]	3 tsp	4 tsp	4 tsp	5 tsp	5 tsp	6 tsp
Discretionary calorie allowance[8]	165	171	171	132	195	267
Calorie Level[1]	**2,200**	**2,400**	**2,600**	**2,800**	**3,000**	**3,200**
Fruits[2]	2 cups	2 cups	2 cups	2.5 cups	2.5 cups	2.5 cups
Vegetables[3]	3 cups	3 cups	3.5 cups	3.5 cups	4 cups	4 cups
Grains[4]	7 oz–eq	8 oz–eq	9 oz–eq	10 oz–eq	10 oz–eq	10 oz–eq
Meat and Beans[5]	6 oz–eq	6.5 oz–eq	6.5 oz–eq	7 oz–eq	7 oz–eq	7 oz–eq
Milk[6]	3 cups	3 cups	3 cups	3 cups	3 cups	3 cups
Oils[7]	6 tsp	7 tsp	8 tsp	8 tsp	10 tsp	11 tsp
Discretionary calorie allowance[8]	290	362	410	426	512	648

1. **Calorie Levels** are set across a wide range to accommodate the needs of different individuals. The attached table "Estimated Daily Calorie Needs" can be used to help assign individuals to the food intake pattern at a particular calorie level.
2. **Fruit Group** includes all fresh, frozen, canned, and dried fruits and fruit juices. In general, 1 cup of fruit or 100% fruit juice, or 1/2 cup of dried fruit can be considered as 1 cup from the fruit group.
3. **Vegetable Group** includes all fresh, frozen, canned, and dried vegetables and vegetable juices. In general, 1 cup of raw or cooked vegetables or vegetable juice, or 2 cups of raw leafy greens can be considered as 1 cup from the vegetable group.

Vegetable Subgroup Amounts Are Per Week

Calorie Level	1,000	1,200	1,400	1,600	1,800	2,000
Dark green veg.	1 c/wk	1.5 c/wk	1.5 c/wk	2 c/wk	3 c/wk	3 c/wk
Orange veg.	.5 c/wk	1 c/wk	1 c/wk	1.5 c/wk	2 c/wk	2 c/wk
Legumes	.5 c/wk	1 c/wk	1 c/wk	2.5 c/wk	3 c/wk	3 c/wk
Starchy veg.	1.5 c/wk	2.5 c/wk	2.5 c/wk	2.5 c/wk	3 c/wk	3 c/wk
Other veg.	3.5 c/wk	4.5 c/wk	4.5 c/wk	5.5 c/wk	6.5 c/wk	6.5 c/wk
Calorie Level	**2,200**	**2,400**	**2,600**	**2,800**	**3,000**	**3,200**
Dark green veg.	3 c/wk	3 c/wk	3 c/wk	3 c/wk	3 c/wk	3 c/wk
Orange veg.	2 c/wk	2 c/wk	2.5 c/wk	2.5 c/wk	2.5 c/wk	2.5 c/wk
Legumes	3 c/wk	3 c/wk	3.5 c/wk	3.5 c/wk	3.5 c/wk	3.5 c/wk
Starchy veg.	6 c/wk	6 c/wk	7 c/wk	7 c/wk	9 c/wk	9 c/wk
Other veg.	7 c/wk	7 c/wk	8.5 c/wk	8.5 c/wk	10 c/wk	10 c/wk

4. **Grains Group** includes all foods made from wheat, rice, oats, cornmeal, barley, such as bread, pasta, oatmeal, breakfast cereals, tortillas, and grits. In general, 1 slice of bread, 1 cup of ready-to-eat cereal, or 1/2 cup of cooked rice, pasta, or cooked cereal can be considered as 1 ounce equivalent from the grains group. **At least half of all grains consumed should be whole grains.**
5. **Meat and Beans Group** in general, 1 ounce of tofu, tempeh, lean meat, poultry, or fish, 1 egg, 1 Tbsp. peanut butter, 1/4 cup cooked dry beans, or 1/2 ounce of nuts or seeds can be considered as 1 ounce equivalent from the meat and beans group. Keep in mind beans will also provide fiber.
6. **Milk Group** includes all fluid milk products (including soy, almond, and brown rice milks) and foods made from milk that retain their calcium content, such as yogurt and cheese (and soy, cashew, almond cheese as well). Foods made from milk that have little to no calcium, such as cream cheese, cream, and butter, are not part of the group. Most milk group choices should be fat-free or low-fat. In general, 1 cup of milk or yogurt, 1 1/2 ounces of natural cheese, or 2 ounces of processed cheese can be considered as 1 cup from the milk group. Keep in mind dark greens are the most absorbable form of calcium and can be eaten instead of any milk, if milk is not desired.
7. **Oils** include fats from many different plants and from fish that are liquid at room temperature, such as canola, corn, olive, soybean, and sunflower oil. Some foods are naturally high in oils, like nuts, olives, some fish, and avocados. Foods that are mainly oil include mayonnaise, certain salad dressings, and soft margarine.
8. **Discretionary Calorie Allowance** is the remaining amount of calories in a food intake pattern after accounting for the calories needed for all food groups—using forms of foods that are fat-free or low-fat and with no added sugars.

MyPyramid Estimated Daily Calorie Needs

To determine which food intake pattern to use for an individual, the following chart gives an estimate of individual calorie needs. The calorie range for each age/sex group is based on physical activity level, from sedentary to active.

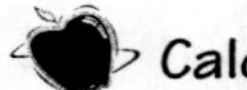 Calorie Range

	Sedentary	*Active*
Children		
2–3 years	1,000	1,400
Females		
4–8 years	1,200	1,800
9–13	1,600	2,200
14–18	1,800	2,400
19–30	2,000	2,400
31–50	1,800	2,200
51+	1,600	2,200
Males		
4–8 years	1,400	2,000
9–13	1,800	2,600
14–18	2,200	3,200
19–30	2,400	3,000
31–50	2,200	3,000
51+	2,000	2,800

Sedentary means a lifestyle that includes only the light physical activity associated with typical day-to-day life.

Active means a lifestyle that includes physical activity equivalent to walking more than 3 miles per day at 3 to 4 miles per hour, in addition to the light physical activity associated with typical day-to-day life.

MyPyramid Tips

MyPyramid Dietary Tips for Busy Schedules that may help you use the guide appropriately and come closer to meeting the guidelines:

- Picture the MyPyramid when you are planning your menu for the day.
- Prepare your lunch the night before—make it a habit and soon it will take only 5 minutes to prep everyone's lunch.
- Plan a sandwich whenever possible—they are hearty and will satisfy you longer than a yogurt or piece of fruit alone. Think of your favorite 4–5 healthful sandwiches, make sure the ingredients are purchased for the whole week, and then prepping is the quick part. Our family favorites are almond butter/jam or baked tofu with mustard/tomato/lettuce, or tofu egg salad (ready-to-spread from Trader Joe's) or an Avocado/Soy Cheese/Veggie sandwich. All are on whole grain bread (Trader Joe's Whole Wheat or House of Bread Dakota are good).
- With the sandwich as the main lunch food, a piece of fruit (or two), whole grain or nut snack (crackers, pretzels, walnuts nut mix etc.), and ready-to-eat carrots can round off a wonderfully healthful lunch.
- Take leftovers from the previous night's dinner whenever available.
- Make weekly dinner plans with each night of the week representing a specific type of dinner. For example, pasta night is Tuesday and Bean Burrito night is Thursday, Saturday is Italian night, etc. This saves the panic of "what are we going to have for dinner tonight?" and helps to establish a theme for the meal from which to build.
- Allow enough time for breakfast at some point in your day even if it is after you arrive at work. Replacing breakfast with coffee tells your fasting body that you are going to raise its blood sugar levels artificially with caffeine. Skipping breakfast and starving in the morning is actually detrimental to weight loss.
- If including veggies during the day is difficult, then try for your minimal cups of veggies at dinnertime. One cup of steamed broccoli and carrots and a cup of salad greens meet your minimal vegetable servings for the day, but try for a colorful salad such as dark greens, red bell pepper, purple onions, orange carrots, yellow apples, with some raisins and walnuts on top with an olive oil-based dressing.
- Try for your minimal fruits either as part of breakfast (banana and O.J.) or for a snack or included in the dinner salad.
- Try for at least 2-grain oz. each in your three meals. If your recommended grain amount is 9 oz., then try for at least 3 oz. in each.
- If you are meeting your whole grain, veggie, and fruit amounts, then protein needs will likely be met, but including two servings of 2–3 oz. of concentrated protein daily will ensure this (legumes, tofu, nuts, seeds, egg whites, low fat dairy, lean meats).
- Choose calcium-rich nuts, seeds, dark green veggies, fortified O.J. and fortified soy and rice milks in addition to dairy foods (choose dairy foods only if you are not intolerant or allergic).

The **Mediterranean Diet Pyramid** was the first pyramid developed by Oldways Preservation and Trust and the Harvard School of Public Health. It is based on healthful diets in the Mediterranean where disease rates are low.

The Traditional Healthy Asian Diet Pyramid

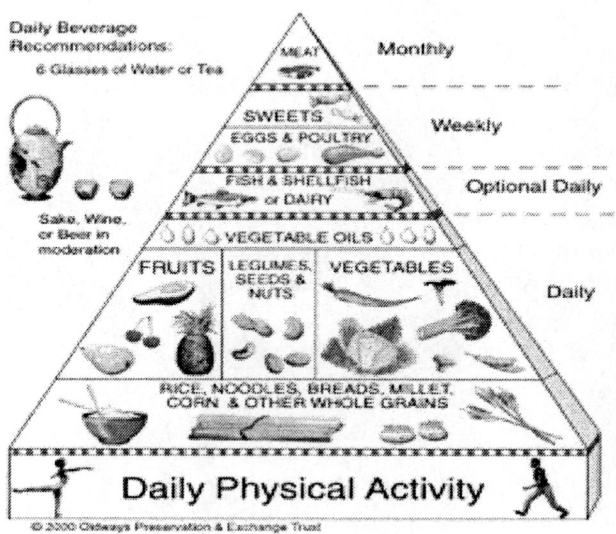

The Traditional Healthy Mediterranean Diet Pyramid

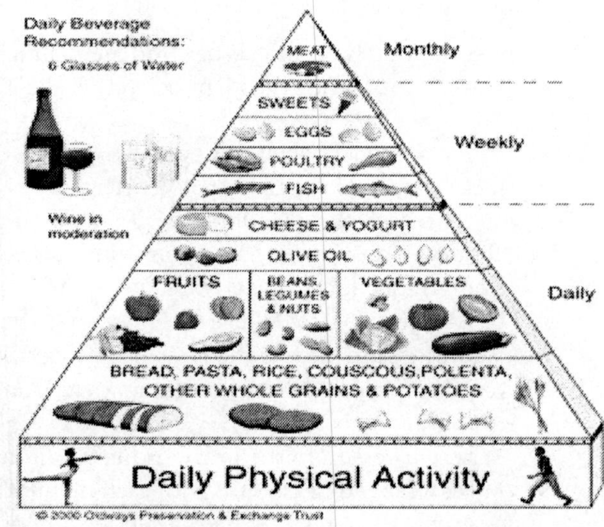

Oldways next developed the **Asian Diet Pyramid**, once again to depict healthful Asian diets where disease rates are low.

Oldways next developed the **Latin American Diet Pyramid**, once again to depict healthful Latin American diets where disease rates are low.

Oldways then developed the **Traditional Healthy Vegetarian Diet Pyramid**, once again to depict healthful Vegetarian diets where disease rates are low.

The Traditional Healthy Vegetarian Diet Pyramid

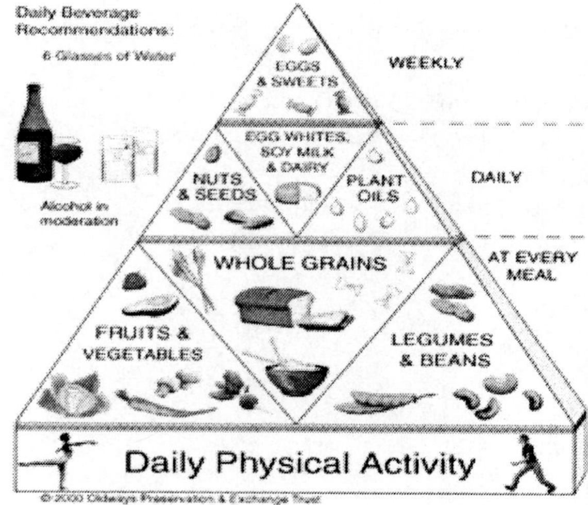

The Traditional Healthy Latin American Diet Pyramid

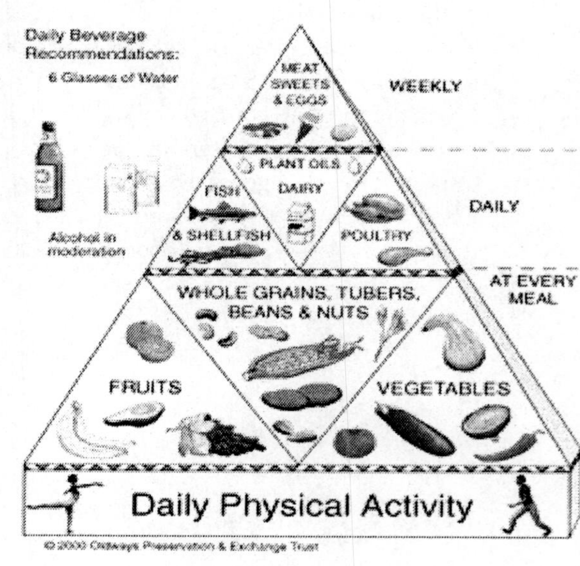

I designed a food guide that would combine the best of every guide along with practical nutrition guidelines, would meet the DRIs, emphasize the most nutrient dense anti-disease phytochemical-rich foods, and promote whole foods. The guide is called **The Healthful House of Food and Fit-**

Focus on the *house* for optimal Wholesome Nutrition!

Roof Additions are *optional*.

Eat **fish** 1–2x/week if you are not a vegetarian.

Choose **non-fat dairy** if you desire dairy.

Choose **egg whites** if you desire eggs.

Choose **lean poultry** over high-fat meats.

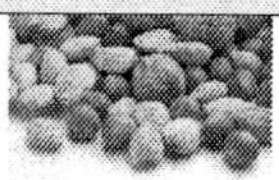

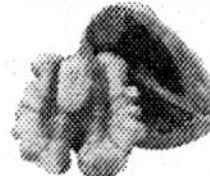

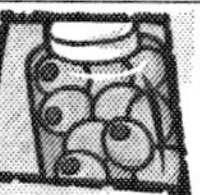

Include small amounts of *Nuts, Seeds, and Healthful Oils* (olive oil and omega-3 fatty acid rich flax seed and walnuts.)

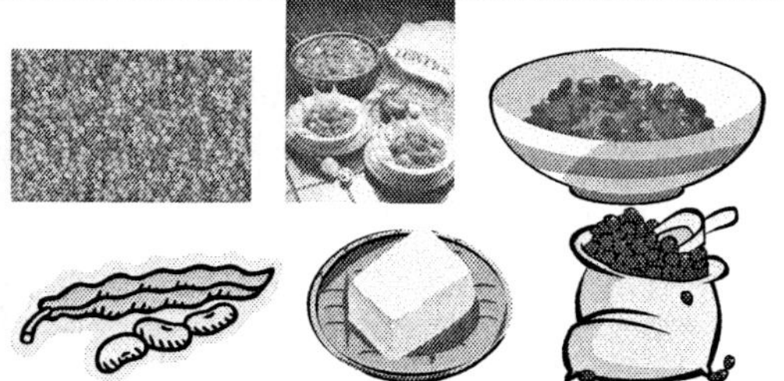

Choose 2–3 servings per day of *Plant Proteins* totaling 50–90 grams per day when added to other foods. (Total depends upon weight and activity.)

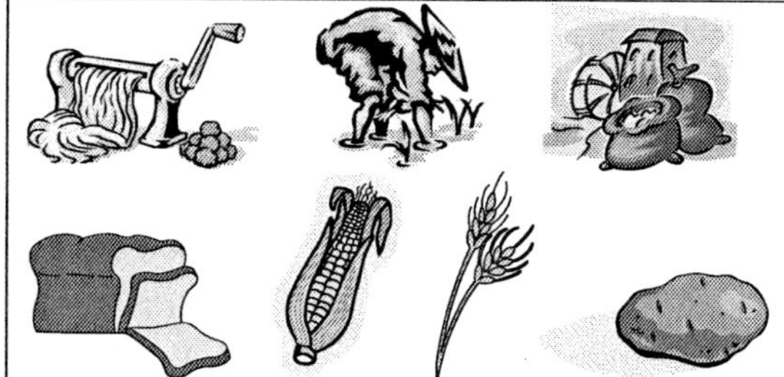

Choose 6–11 servings per day of *High Fiber Whole Grains and Starchy Vegetables*, adding carbohydrates with those in fruits, veggies, and legumes for a total of 300–700 grams daily, depending on total activity.

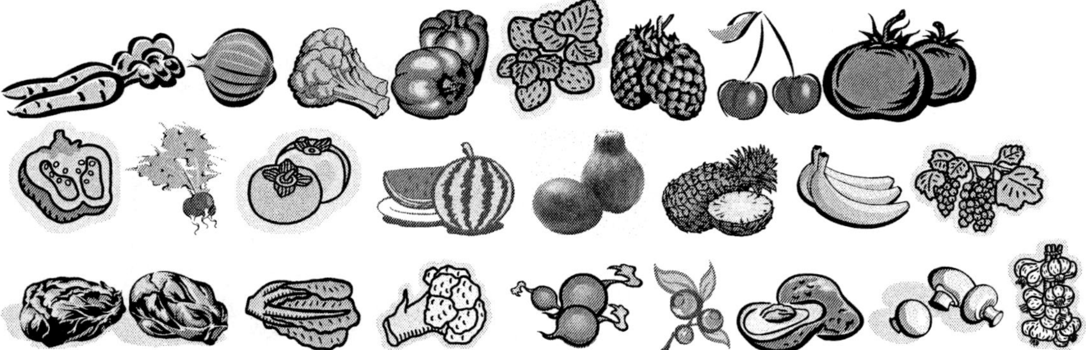

Choose 7–11 servings per day of *Phytonutrient-Rich Fruits and Vegetables* of all rainbow colors.

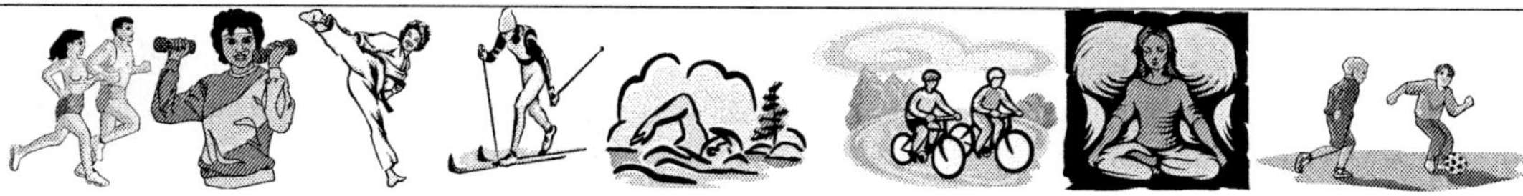

Build a foundation of *Daily Physical Activities* of stretching, cardio exercise, muscle work and recreation.

ness because it also highly encourages all of the aspects of health-related physical fitness (flexibility, muscular endurance, cardiovascular endurance and strength) as the foundation of the house.

Important points about the House are as follows:

- **Build a foundation of Daily Physical Activities of stretching, cardio exercise, muscle work and recreation.**
  - Physical Activity reduces chances of all causes of death.
  - Participate in flexibility, strength, muscular endurance, and cardiovascular endurance activities.
- **Choose 7–11 servings per day of Phytonutrient-Rich Fruits and Vegetables of all rainbow colors.**
  - Choose a variety such as red (tomatoes), orange (tangerines), yellow (grapefruit), green (broccoli), blue (blueberries), white (garlic) and yellow-green (avocado).
  - Each color category covers a different set of powerful phytochemicals.
- **Choose 6–11 servings per day of High Fiber Whole Grains and Starchy Vegetables, adding carbohydrates with those in fruits, veggies, and legumes for a total of 300–700 grams daily, depending on total activity.**
  - The average person needs about 300 grams of carbohydrates daily to reach 60% of Calories from carbohydrate in a 2000 Calorie diet.
  - The phytonutrient-rich fruits and veggies may contribute 1/3 of these needs and legumes may contribute some more.
  - Use a diet analysis program to check your carbohydrate intake when all of the House categories are added together.
  - Limit refined grains that have had their fiber and nutrients removed.
  - No simple sugars have been listed in the House, but unrefined simple sugars such as honey, fruit juice, and pure maple syrup may be eaten sparingly (less than 10% of total Calories) when nutrient needs have been met.
  - Athletes needing 700 grams of carbohydrate daily will have room for more simple sugars.
- **Choose 2–3 servings per day of Plant Proteins totaling 50–90 grams per day when added to other foods. (Total depends upon weight and activity.)**
  - The veggie and fruit and whole grain categories will contribute protein so be sure to add those together with this category or use a diet analysis program to check total protein intake.
  - Plant proteins such as tofu, lentils, and tempeh have many health benefits over animal proteins such as phytonutrients and fiber.
- **Include small amounts of Nuts, Seeds, and Healthful Oils (olive oil and omega-3 fatty acid-rich flax seed and walnuts).**
  - Unsaturated non-hydrogenated fats, especially omega-3-rich (linolenic acids) benefit the heart by lowering cholesterol.
  - Fat is concentrated in Calories so be careful not to eat huge amounts.
  - Blend fresh organic flax seed in the blender and add to smoothies or sprinkle on cereals or healthful desserts (i.e., Soy Dream ice cream)
- **The optional additions are for those wishing to consume some animal foods:**
  - Eat *fish* 1–2x/week if you are not vegetarian (it contains omega-3 fatty acids)
  - Choose *non-fat dairy* if you desire dairy (dairy fat is high in saturated fat and cholesterol)
  - Choose *egg whites* if you desire eggs (the yellow contains the cholesterol)
  - Choose *lean poultry* over high fat meats (lean turkey has the least fat)

Exchange Lists for Choosing Foods

The final tool discussed in this chapter for designing diets is Exchange Lists. The American Dietetics Association and the American Diabetes Association created an exchange list system that has been changed over the years to accommodate new foods and new research on nutrition. People attempting to lose weight and athletes may use the exchange list system to make day-to-day meal planning easier than calculating each of your energy nutrients daily.

The exchange lists are designed to ensure that you get a specific amount of Calories and Energy Nutrients (Fat, Carb and Protein) whereas you are able to choose which foods you want to eat as long as you adhere to the serving amounts and the number of servings (exchanges) from each category. The system does not ensure that you will make the most nutritious choices for vitamins and minerals (i.e., It does not distinguish between white bread and 7-grain bread). Some programs are based on higher fat or protein diets so be sure to choose an exchange program that meets your personal needs.

The following chart gives the six exchange list categories, their composition of energy nutrients, and samples of the exchanges amounts of selected foods:

Exchange List Categories/Composition of Energy Nutrients/ Sample Amounts of Foods

Category	*Energy Nutrient Breakdown*	*One exchange equals:*
Starch (80 kcal)	15 grams carbohydrate 3 grams protein 0–1 grams fat	1 slice bread, tortilla, or roll ½ cup cooked pasta, barley, cooked cereal, rice milk ⅓ cup cooked brown rice, couscous, baked beans ½ cup corn, peas, yams, winter squash, lentils, beans 1 small (3 oz.) baked potato ½ bagel, English muffin, bun, pita ¾ cup dry flaked cereal 3 cups air-popped popcorn or ¾ oz. pretzels 2 rice cakes or 2–5 whole-wheat crackers, no fat ¼ cup low-fat granola, grape nuts, millet, muesli 3 Tbs. wheat germ
Vegetable (25 kcal)	5 grams carbohydrate 2 grams protein 0 grams fat	½ cup cooked vegetables or vegetable juice 1 cup raw vegetables
Fruit (60 kcal)	15 grams carbohydrate 0 grams protein 0 grams fat	1 small to medium fresh fruit ½ cup fresh or canned fruit (no sugar) or fruit juice ¾–1 cup berries or melon ¼ cup dried fruit (8 dried apricot halves, 2 medium figs) 17 small grapes 2 Tbs. raisins ½ papaya, grapefruit, mango
Protein—Legumes, Meats, Cheeses (55–100 kcal)	0 grams carbohydrate 7 grams protein 1–8 grams fat (depending on whether food is very lean, lean, medium fat or high fat)	4 oz. tofu ½ cup cooked beans, peas, lentils (count as one starch also) 2 Tbs. nut butter 1 small tofu, turkey or chicken dog 1 oz. processed sandwich meats and meat analogs (vegetarian version of baloney and deli slices) 1 egg 1 oz. poultry, fish, beef, pork, etc. 1 oz. cheese
Milk (90–150 kcal)	12 grams carbohydrate 8 grams protein 0–8 grams fat (depending on amount of fat in milk)	1 cup milk (fat varies from 0 in nonfat to 8 grams in whole milk) 1 cup yogurt (fat varies from 0–8 grams) Soy milk similar in energy nutrients to low-fat cow milk
Fat (45 kcal)	0 grams carbohydrate 0 grams protein 5 grams fat	1 tsp. oil, margarine, butter, mayonnaise 1 Tbs. cream cheese, cream, nuts ⅛ medium avocado (see Chapter 5 for best fats—canola oil, olive oil, nuts, seeds)

There is also a Free Foods List with items that do not contain any significant amount of energy nutrients; but some may be high in sodium. Examples are lemon juice, coffee, herbal tea, mustard, soy sauce, vinegar, pickles, garlic, bouillon, and salsa.

Suggested Daily Meal Guidelines Using the Food Exchange List System

Number of Exchanges from each Category for Specific Caloric Intakes

Daily Calories	***~1500***	***~2000***	***~2500***	***~3000***	***~3500***	***~4000***
Starch	8	12	16	19	22	26
Vegetable	6	6	7	7	8	9
Fruit	4	4	5	6	8	9
Nonfat, 1%, or soy milk	2	2	2	3	3	3
Lean protein	2	3	3	3	4	4
Fat	5	6	7	9	11	13

The above suggestions consist of about 62–65% carbohydrate/13-17% protein/20% fat. The calories are estimated a little high to add for some possible fat in the starch category. The protein is slightly higher than needed.

The following is a sample menu using the exchange list system:

Menu is:
1500 Calories
63% carb (234 gms)
18% protein (66 gms)
19% fat (31 grams)

Total Exchanges Chosen Per Day:
9 starches
4 fruit
6 vegetable
2 high proteins (lean)
2 nonfat milk
5 fats

Breakfast	
1 cup bran cereal, flakes	2 starch
1 banana	2 fruit
1/2 cup applesauce	1 fruit
1 cup skim milk (or soy)	1 milk
Lunch	
2 slices WW bread	2 starch
1 oz. turkey (no skin)	1 high protein
Tomato/lettuce/onion	1/2 vegetable
1 tsp. mustard	Free
1 tsp. nonfat mayo	Free
1 small whole baked potato	1 starch
1 tsp. nonhydrogenated margarine	1 fat
6 oz. vegetable juice	1.5 vegetable
Dinner	
1 cup black beans, cooked	2 starch, 1 high protein
1 cup chopped tomato, spinach, onions	1 vegetable
2 WW tortillas with no lard	2 starch
1/2 avocado	4 fat
Fresh salsa	Free
1 cup cooked broccoli	2 vegetable
1 cup salad (greens, carrots, red pepper)	1 vegetable
AM snack	
4 medium apricots	1 fruit
PM snack	
1 cup nonfat yogurt or soy yogurt	1 nonfat dairy

Exchange Lists can very helpful, but the ultimate tool for helping you to meet nutrient needs is to assess, evaluate, then adjust your diet with the help of a computer dietary analysis program. The diet analysis program packaged with your book can help you to take all of this information about essential nutrient requirements and design a personalized program for your individual needs. The details of how to go about assessing your diet will be covered later in this book. This process is ongoing and an important ingredient in achieving optimal nutrition for a lifetime.

chapter 3

Human Body Systems and Digestion

The human body is a complex organism made up of many units from the millions of cellular components to the systems working together in unison to keep it functioning. Cells combine to form tissues, which combine to form organs, which combine to form body systems. Every cell requires nutrients and energy in the form of adenosine triphosphate (ATP).

The Systems of the Human Body

Many systems in the body work together to help each other function properly and to keep the human body working as a unit:

- The **circulatory** system involves pulmonary, systemic, portal, and lymphatic circulation.
- The **cardiovascular** system is the heart (cardio) pumping blood to the lungs and the network of arteries, capillaries, and veins all working to move nutrients and oxygen by way of blood to the body's cells.
- The **respiratory** system represents the tissues and organs involved in breathing, such as the bronchioles and lungs.
- The **endocrine** system is the regulatory system that contains the glands thyroid, adrenal, pituitary and the pancreas, ovaries, and testes that secrete hormones to balance, control, and regulate other substances in the body (such as the pancreas secreting insulin to regulate blood glucose).
- The **urinary** system includes the kidneys, ureter, bladder, and urethra that remove waste products and regulate blood acid-base balance. Proper function of this system is determined by the cardiovascular system, fluid intake, and drug use.
- The **lymphatic** system contains lymph and immune cells. It allows the passage of large particles such as large fats, and this system eventually empties into veins leading to the heart.
- The **nervous** system is also a regulatory system involving the central nervous system (brain and the spinal cord) and the peripheral nervous system that branches out to the organs. Neurons respond to electrical and chemical signals to allow the nervous system to function.
- The **immune** system is the body's defense against invading pathogens by way of the skin, intestinal cells, and white blood cells. It is a sensitive indicator of the body's nutritional status. Your immune system can be strengthened with rest, reduced stress, moderate exercise, and functional nutrition such as phytonutrients and antioxidants in colorful fruits and vegetables and herbs such as echinacea and goldenseal.
- The **excretory** system is responsible for the removal of waste products via the urine, skin (perspiration), and the lungs (CO_2).
- The "**storage** system" allows the body to retain nutrition and energy in the form of adipose tissue (fat), glycogen in liver and muscle, calcium in bones, amino acids in the blood, and vitamins and minerals in the liver.
- The **digestive** system works intricately with these other systems; the rest of this chapter will focus on the digestive system parts and their functions and disorders.

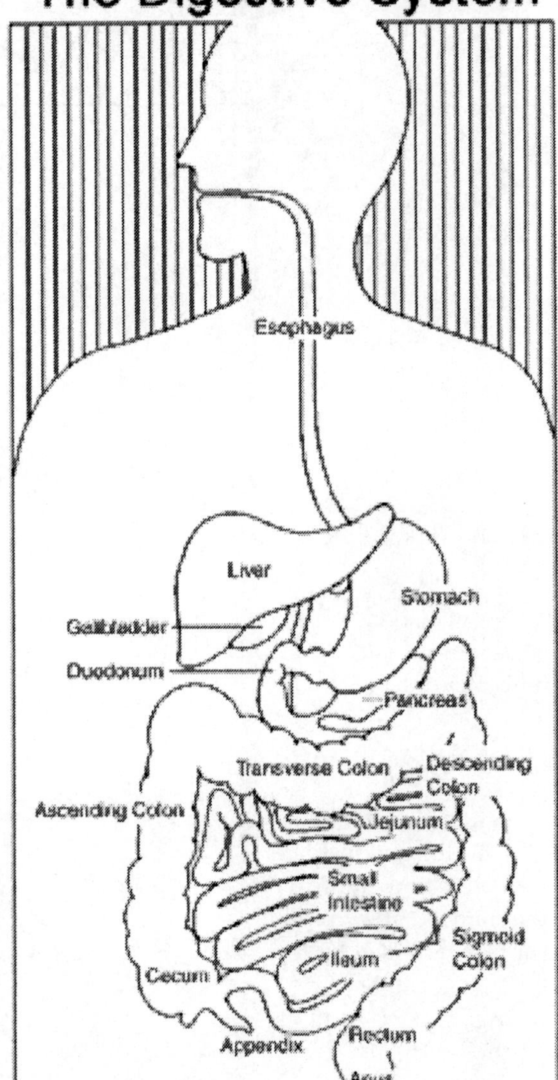

The GI Tract

The first part of the digestive system is the mouth, which is used for mastication, produces saliva that lubricates the food for easier swallowing, and provides the enzyme amylase to begin starch breakdown. The tongue has taste receptors and aids in chewing. There are also enzymes active in infants that help break down fatty acids, which is important with their 50% fat diet of mother's milk.

The food then moves into the **esophagus**, which is a long tube that with gravity and lubricating mucus pushes food to the stomach by way of peristalsis. **Peristalsis** is a contracting and relaxing of the smooth involuntary muscle that occurs throughout the gastrointestinal tract. Where the esophagus meets the stomach is the **esophageal sphincter** that controls the flow of food into the stomach. If stomach acids come back through the sphincter into the esophagus, then heartburn occurs.

The food then enters the **stomach,** where some protein digestion occurs. The stomach secretes acid, enzymes, and an intrinsic factor to help food churn into a liquid mass called chyme. There is a mucous layer preventing the stomach from digesting itself (autodigestion). Depending on the type of food, the stomach can hold food for 2–4 hours and has a capacity of about 4 cups. The **pyloric sphincter** controls the flow of the chyme into the small intestine. Specific roles of the stomach acid are that it destroys the activity of protein, activates digestive enzymes, partially digests dietary protein, assists in calcium absorption, and makes dietary minerals soluble for absorption.

The food substance then moves to the next section of the GI tract which is the **small intestine** where most digestion and absorption occurs. The small intestine digests 95% of the total meal. There are three parts: duodenum (10 inches), jejunum (4 feet), and ileum (5 feet). The muscle of the small intestine contracts and the walls are folded. **Villi** projections are located on the folds, and absorptive cells are located on the villi that increase the intestinal surface area 600 times. Rapid cell turnover occurs on the surface of the small intestine. These intestinal cells have mucosal membranes, act as barriers to invading microbes, and have immunoglobulins that produce immune bodies. A deficiency of nutrients can cause these cells not to function properly, therefore leading to absorption problems. Consuming human milk as an infant instead of artificial infant formula develops the entire flora of the intestine for a lifetime, which can positively affect one's immunity to disease, especially intestinal illnesses.

The next section of the tract is the **large intestine (colon)** and is about 3½ feet in length and typically referred to in three parts: ascending colon, transverse colon, and descending colon. It contains bacterial flora, but no villi or enzymes are present, and little digestion occurs. There is some absorption of water, some minerals, and vitamins and the indigestible food stuff combines with water for the formation of feces for elimination. The rectum holds the stool remains, stimulates elimination, and uses muscle contractions for elimination. **Anal sphincters** control the final step in digestion, with the final sphincter being voluntary (most of the time and after infancy).

The four sphincters of the digestive tract are the lower **esophagus sphincter, pyloric sphincter, ileocecal sphincter,** and the **anal sphincters**.

The Accessory Organs

The accessory organs (pancreas, gallbladder, and liver) play a vital role in the functioning of the digestive system and the human body, although they are not part of the tract that the food flows through. The **liver**'s main function in digestion is to produce bile that will be stored in the gall bladder and released when needed via the bile duct into the small intestine for emulsifying fats. The liver also transports the nutrients via the blood once they have been absorbed and processes them before returning them to the bloodstream. The liver is the main site of metabolism. The liver plays many roles in metabolism including deanimating proteins, storing glycogen, detoxifying alcohol and drugs, and making cholesterol. The **pancreas** manufactures digestive enzymes, produces glucagon and insulin, secretes pancreatic juices, and makes bicarbonate needed to neutralize the acidic chyme from the stomach. The **gallbladder** stores bile until it is needed. Although the accessory organs are not actually part of the GI tract, they are essential for digestive system functioning.

Digestive Disorders

There are over 100 digestive system disorders/diseases. A few common disorders follow.

Ulcers

Symptoms:	Pain ~2 hrs after eating
Causes:	*Helicobacter pylori* Excessive use of aspirin Excessive acid production Stress Stomach loses its mucous protection
Do:	Eat regular meals, refrain from smoking, limit use of aspirin, limit spices, add fiber, and lose weight.

Heartburn *or gastroesophageal reflux disease (GERD)*

Symptoms:	Gnawing pain in the upper chest
Causes:	Movement of acid from the stomach into the esophagus
Do:	Eat smaller, more frequent meals, low in fat, wait 2 hours before lying down, refrain from smoking, lose excess weight, limit spicy foods, limit citrus.

Constipation

Symptoms:	Difficult or infrequent bowel movement
Causes:	Slow motility, medication, and supplements of calcium/iron Feces stay in the large intestine longer Ignore normal urges to defecate
Do:	Eat plenty of dietary fiber, drink more fluids, regular physical activity, relaxation.

Hemorrhoids

Symptoms:	Swollen veins of the rectum and anus Intense pressure and straining Pain, itching, bleeding
Causes:	Obesity, pregnancy, prolonged sitting, violent coughing, low-fiber diet
Do:	Eat a high-fiber diet, fluids, warm compresses.

Irritable Bowel Syndrome

Symptoms:	Cramps, gassiness, bloating, irregular bowel function
Cause:	Altered intestinal peristalsis and decreased pain threshold
Do:	An individualized elimination diet, moderate caffeine, low fat, small meals, stress reduction.

Diarrhea

Symptoms:	Increased fluidity, frequency, or amount of bowel movement
Cause:	Infection in the intestine (bacteria and viruses cause the intestinal cells to secrete fluid)
Do:	Consume plenty of fluid during the affected stage.

The metabolism of the nutrients from absorption to releasing energy for the cells to create muscular work will be covered in chapter 15.

chapter 4

Carbohydrates—The Preferred Fuel

Carbohydrates are the preferred source of energy for all body functions and muscular exertions, and they are necessary to assist other foods in digestion, assimilation, and elimination. Carbohydrates differ so greatly from one to the next that to label all carbohydrates as "bad" or "good" would represent a total misunderstanding of food and nutrients. Not all carbohydrates are created equal.

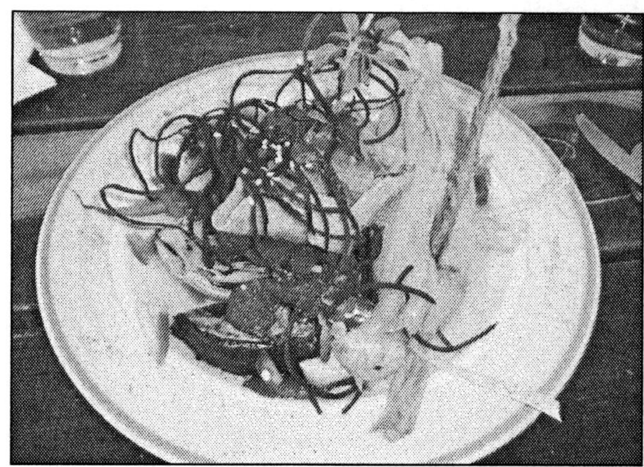

A Gourmet Dinner Rich in Complex Carbohydrates

What Are Carbohydrates?

Carbohydrates can be classified into **simple** or **complex**, depending on the length of the saccharide chain. When the term *simple* is used, it is referring to the single or double molecule of sugar (the **monosaccharides** and the **disaccharides**). Examples of monosaccharides in the diet are **glucose**, **fructose**, and **galactose**. These monosaccharides bond to form the disaccharides. Examples of disaccharides in the diet are **sucrose**, **lactose**, and **maltose**. A glucose molecule and another glucose molecule form maltose. A glucose and a galactose molecule form milk sugar, which is lactose. A glucose and a fructose (fruit sugar) molecule form sucrose (table sugar). Long chains of sugar or glucose units are polysaccharides such as amylose. **Fiber** is also a form of complex carbohydrate. Food examples of simple carbohydrates are sugar, honey, fructose, glucose, corn syrup, brown sugar, and foods made with these sweeteners such as cookies, cakes, pies, candy, ice cream, and soda pop. Simple sugars are sweet. Examples of complex carbohydrates or polysaccharides are grains, vegetables, fruits, peas, and beans. If carbohydrates have had their bran kernel and germ removed, then this great loss of fiber and nutrients leaves them "refined" and of much lesser value nutritionally. When grains are "enriched," then these vital components have been removed and only a few nutrients have been replaced.

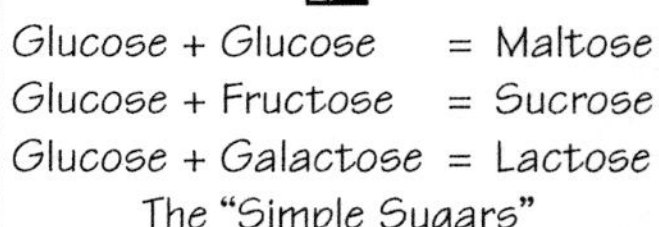

Glucose + Glucose = Maltose
Glucose + Fructose = Sucrose
Glucose + Galactose = Lactose
The "Simple Sugars"

Consume Healthful Carbohydrates

Several problems may occur with the consumption of too many simple refined sugary "sweet" carbohydrates such as the following.

- **Unstable blood sugar levels**
- **Diabetes and hypoglycemia**
- **Obesity and weight problems**
- **Rapid pulse and trembling**
- **Headaches, anxiety, and confusion**
- **Tooth decay**
- **Insomnia**
- **Nervousness and depression**
- **Inadequate nutrient intake by replacing nutritious foods with the "empty" caloric simple refined carbohydrates. "Empty" meaning that the Calories are not filled with any nutritive value.**

Healthful sources of unrefined wholesome complex carbohydrates are the following.

Products that have whole grains as the first ingredient:
Whole-grain waffles
Whole-grain cereals
Whole wheat bread
Whole wheat tortillas
Whole wheat pasta

Whole grains:
Oats
Barley
Millet
Rye
Triticale
Bulgur
Kamut
Brown rice

All fresh veggies and fruits:
Fruits also have the natural simple sugar fructose.

Legumes:
Lentils
Split peas
Beans (black, white, kidney, garbanzo, adzuki, etc.)

Less-healthful complex carbohydrates are the refined ones such as white bread, white noodles, and enriched cereals. Specific ideas for adding and preparing healthful carbohydrates to your personal dietary program are given in detail in chapter 14, "Consumer Nutrition." A high-carbohydrate diet that contains these wholesome unrefined complex types is also rich in fiber, rich in vitamins and minerals, rich in phytochemicals, has essential fatty acids, is rich in antioxidants, and promotes satiety.

Therefore the health benefits of a diet high in these complex carbohydrate nutrient-rich foods is that it can prevent coronary heart disease, prevent certain cancers, lower cholesterol, prevent hemorrhoids, prevent diverticulitis, prevent appendicitis, and reduce the risk of obesity.

Carbohydrate Digestion, Absorption, and Functions

Carbohydrates are digested in the body with the help of enzymes that split polysaccharides and disaccharides into monosaccharides, which are the form that can be absorbed. **Salivary amylase** is a carbohydrate-digesting enzyme that is released by the salivary glands. The pancreas releases **pancreatic amylase** that continues this breakdown toward monosaccharides. The surface of the small intestine will contribute additional enzymes to complete the breakdown, and then the monosaccharides are absorbed through the wall of the small intestine in the **jejunum** section. Here they will travel to the liver, where they will all be converted to glucose for energy or storage. If someone has a lack of the lactase enzyme that splits apart lactose (milk sugar), then the lactose may remain in the small intestine and become fermented, causing serious gastrointestinal pain. This condition (**lactose intolerance**) is very common in people of African, Mexican, Asian, Native American, and Philippine backgrounds. It commonly occurs after the natural age of weaning of mother's milk in those societies (beyond 4 or so years), so babies and young children do not commonly have lactose intolerance. Cow's milk is not a good source of calcium for individuals with lactose intolerance.

Once the monosaccharides are converted to glucose after being digested and absorbed, they have many functions in the human body, including **blood glucose maintenance** (80 Calories), **glycogen storage in the liver** (400 Calories), **muscle glycogen storage** (1400–1800 Calories), and serve as the primary brain fuel. Carbohydrates are essential for athletes, especially endurance athletes, and when depleted in the liver and muscles are one of the leading causes of fatigue.

Carbohydrate Needs

The government recommends at least **55% of total Calories** come from carbohydrates for the average person. The WHO (World Health Organization) recommends that **70%–80% of total Calories** in the diet be from carbohydrates. Athletes need total carbohydrate grams to be closer to the WHO standard in order to properly store enough fuel for their events, especially for endurance competition. A minimal daily amount of carbohydrates recommended for an athlete is **300 grams**. Most athletes will need **500–700 grams of carbohydrate daily**. Specific carbohydrate charts for active people and athletes are listed in chapter 16.

Fiber Fitness

The average American diet obtains 91% of its Calories from nonfiber types of foods such as meat (20%), refined cereals (20%), visible fats (18%), sugar (17%), milk (12%), eggs (2%), and alcohol (2%). Consequently, the average American diet contains **12 grams of fiber** a day, too little for a healthy colon. The recommendation for a healthy amount of fiber varies between **25–60 grams of fiber** a day. In both agriculturalist and hunter-gathering ancient diets **60–100 grams of fiber** was consumed daily. Both types of fiber, insoluble fiber and soluble fiber, have health benefits such as reduced cholesterol levels, less colon disease, and the promotion of weight control. Some examples of names of fibers naturally found in foods are **hemicelluloses**, **pectin**, and **gums**. The foods with the highest amounts of fiber are **beans**, **legumes**, and **peas**, then whole grain cereals, whole grain flours, and whole grain products, potatoes, and yams. Next highest in fiber after the beans and whole grains are generally most fruits, and vegetables then seeds and nuts. Foods that contain no fiber are meat, milk, eggs, sugar, and alcohol.

In addition to the weight-control benefit and reduced blood cholesterol and colon disease, fiber also benefits health by promoting softer, larger stools and regularity, it slows glucose absorption, and it reduces hemorrhoids and diverticula.

The kernels of grains (such as wheat, barley, oat, rye, corn, rice, triticale) consist of three major parts:

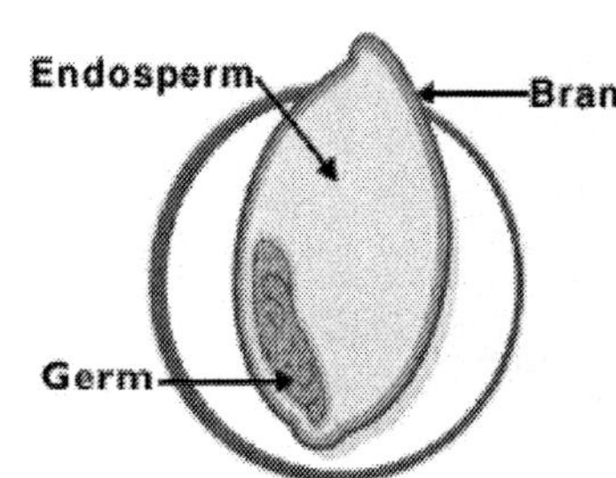

Bran—this is the outer layer of the grain (14%–16% of wheat, 5%–6% of corn)
Endosperm—this is the main part of the grain
Germ—this is the smallest part of the grain

Whole grains contain all three layers of the grain.

Whole-grain cereals provide a rich source of many essential vitamins, minerals, and phytochemicals. The typical whole grain cereal food is:

- Low in saturated fat but has polyunsaturated fats, including omega-3 fatty acids
- Cholesterol free
- High in both soluble and insoluble fiber
- An excellent source of complex carbohydrates
- A significant source of protein
- A good source of B-complex vitamins, including folate
- A good source of many minerals (i.e., iron, magnesium, zinc, and copper)
- A good source of antioxidants, including vitamin E and selenium
- A good source of phytochemicals including phytoestrogens, phytic acid, flavonoids and phytosterols (which can help lower blood cholesterol levels)

Research is currently directing its attention now to whole-grain cereals as being a significant source of these antioxidant phytochemicals, including phytoestrogens. Whole-grain cereals contain many different phytochemicals that researchers have linked to significant health benefits. These phytochemicals include

- **Lignin:** An insoluble fiber phytoestrogen that is a naturally occurring component of plant life that helps provide strength in plants and can lower the risk of coronary heart disease and may protect against hormonally linked diseases such as breast and prostate cancer. Lignins are mostly found in outer layers (such as wheat bran) and are high in flaxseed.
- **Phytic acid:** Reduces the glycemic index of food, which is important for people with diabetes and helps protect against the development of cancer cells in the colon. It was previously thought to be a disadvantage because it binds iron and zinc and makes it unavailable for absorption. It is

now known to act as an important *antioxidant,* which protects the bowel wall from damaging chemical reactions.

- **Saponins, phytosterols, squalene, oryzanol and tocotrienols:** Have been found to lower blood cholesterol.
- **Phenolic compounds**: Have antioxidant effects.

Sugar Substitutes

Although some simple sugars in the diet (up to 10% of Calories) are considered to be harmless, the average American chooses to consume about **24 pounds of artificial sugar substitutes a year**. It is true that most of these substitutes will not promote tooth decay, will not affect blood glucose levels, and are very low Calorie, but the negative effects may outweigh the few positive ones. **Saccharin**, for example, which is 300 times sweeter than sucrose, is known to cause cancer in laboratory animals, and warning labels are required on all foods that contain it. Another artificial sweetener, **aspartame** (Nutrasweet), is 200 times sweeter than sucrose and its safety is extremely controversial. It is believed to increase serotonin levels, which can increase depression. It is definitely not recommended to people with the disorder phenylketonuria (PKU). The newest artificial sweeteners are **acesulfame (Sunette)** and **sucralose (Splenda),** which is found in many Atkins products. Acesulfame is 200 times sweeter than sucrose and not digested by the body. Sucralose is 600 times sweeter than sucrose and has chlorine added to make the body unable to digest it, which has led to many digestive problems such as bloating, cramping, and enlarged organs.

Diabetes and Hypoglycemia

Diabetes is a disease associated with high blood sugar levels (hyperglycemia), insulin control problems, and a series of additional symptoms. Diabetes can go undiagnosed for years and be fatal if not properly controlled. **Type 1** diabetes contributes to 10%–20% of cases and requires one to be insulin dependent. The person that is Type 1 generally has low body fat, severe symptoms, impaired insulin function, and often an early onset of the disease in life. There is a link between feeding artificial milk (cow's milk formula) and regular cow's milk as a baby and Type 1 diabetes. An exclusively breast-fed baby appears to be somewhat protected from Type 1 diabetes. **Type 2** diabetes occurs in about 90% of the cases and is non-insulin-dependent. The person has high body fat, has less symptoms, develops the disease later in life, has lifestyle-related reasons, and can often control the disease by losing weight and exercising.

To diagnose diabetes, one usually receives a lab procedure called the glucose tolerance test, which is one of the diagnostic tools that is measured after a fast. The patient drinks a sugar solution, then his or her blood is tested to check blood sugar levels at half-hour intervals. If the blood sugar rises and does not come back down on its own, it may be an indication of an insulin production problem and diabetes. **Gestational diabetes** is an additional form of diabetes that occurs only during pregnancy, and symptoms go away after the baby is born. Major symptoms of diabetes include excessive urination and thirst, and the results of diabetes can be heart disease, blindness, and other circulatory problems.

The two hormones primarily responsible for regulating the blood sugar levels in the body are insulin and glucagon. Insulin promotes glycogen synthesis, increases glucose uptake by the cells, reduces gluconeogenesis, and essentially lowers the blood glucose. Glucagon breaks down glycogen, enhances gluconeogenesis, and essentially raises blood glucose. The diagram on the following page shows this process of blood sugar regulating with insulin and glucagon.

Hypoglycemia is a condition in which blood sugar levels fall lower than what is considered to be normal. One type of hypoglycemia is **reactive (postprandial)**, and the symptoms, generally after a meal, are fatigue, weakness, confusion, dizziness, irritability, rapid heartbeat, sweating, trembling, hunger, and headaches. **Fasting hypoglycemia** represents symptoms after not eating such as dullness, fatigue, confusion, amnesia, seizures, and unconsciousness. True hypoglycemia is diagnosed by a doctor, but anyone can experience the symptoms of low blood sugar. Some of the reasons for diagnosed hypoglycemia are cancer, pancreatic damage, liver infection and damage, alcohol-induced liver disease, and sugary meals. Some tips for dealing with low blood sugar are eating balanced meals (5–6 each day) of complex carbs, fats, and protein in each meal (breakdown according to individual needs assessed in the diet analysis program), the avoidance of alcohol and caffeine, and to increase exercise and reduce stress in one's life.

The glycemic index that is discussed in many of the faddish low-carb diet books implies that whole foods (i.e., bananas, raisins, carrots, corn, potatoes, pineapple, and watermelon) that have been found to cause a high sugar reaction in your body should always be avoided. However, the testing of these foods is inconclusive, and many of these foods can be eaten with other complex carb/protein/fat foods and *not* cause a reaction. Common sense might be knowing some of these foods and not eating them alone in great quantities if one is sensitive, but remembering that whole fruits, veggies, and grains are the most abundant source of carbohydrate fuel for anyone, including athletes and active people. Carbohydrates are even ergogenic in the sense that performance is greatly hindered without them! Foods that are naturally rich in carbohydrates (vegetable, fruits, whole grains, and legumes) are those foods that are necessary for healthful nutrition for a lifetime!

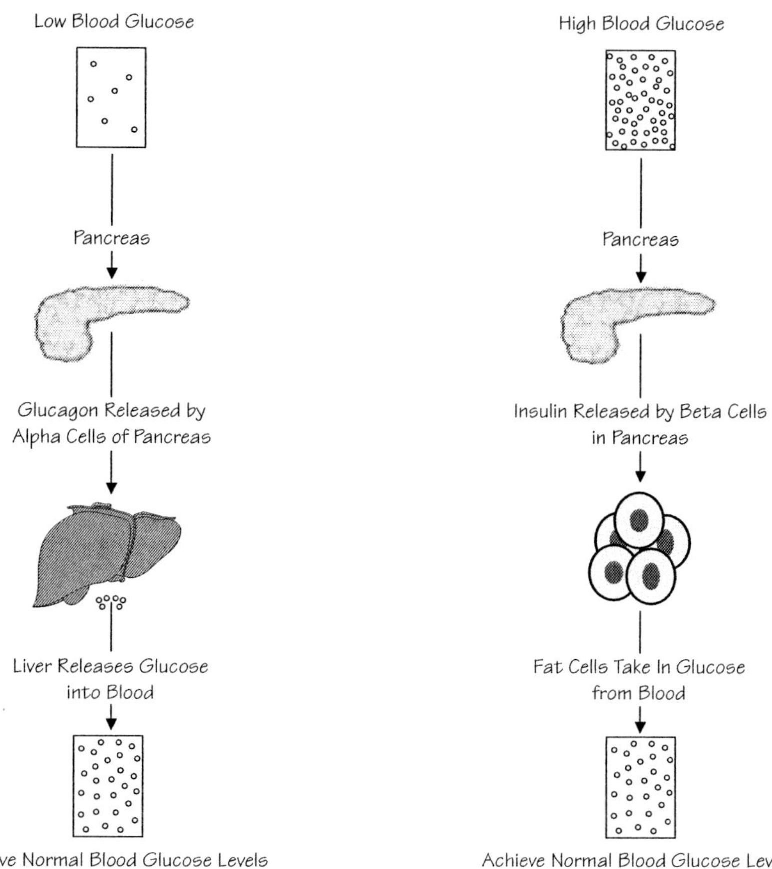

chapter 5

Lipids for Health

All Food Fats Were Not Created Equal!

"Lipids" is the general term for all fats and oils. A lipid is an energy-yielding nutrient that provides 9 Calories per gram. Although fat is the most abused food group in the American diet and most Americans consume 35%–37% of their daily Calories from fat, too much recent attention has been spent promoting nonfat (and often nutrient-poor) diets, when actually a diet moderate in healthful fats and low in harmful fats can promote health, decrease disease, and promote weight loss.

Classifying Lipids

The most common type of food fat (about 90% of all food fats) is a **triglyceride**, which is composed of a **glycerol** and **three fatty acids**. The three fatty acids can either be saturated or unsaturated. The **saturated fatty acids** carry the maximum number of hydrogen atoms in their chemical structure. The **unsaturated fatty acids** have one or more points of unsaturation occurring in their chemical struc-

Type of Fat as a Percentage of Total Fat Content

	Monounsaturated	Polyunsaturated	Saturated
Coconut oil	6	2	92
Milk, butter, cream fat	30[1]	4	66
Cocoa butter	34	3	63[2]
Beef tallow	44	14	52
Palm oil	39	10	51
Lard (pork fat)	41	11	42
Chicken fat	47	23	30
Safflower oil	13	78	9
Sunflower oil	20	69	11
Corn oil	25	62	13
Soybean oil	24	61	15
Cottonseed oil	19	54	27
Fish oil	30	40[3]	20–30
Olive oil[5]	77	9	14
Canola oil (rapeseed)[5]	58	36	6
Peanut oil	48	34	18
Margarine[4]			
Soybean oil stick	49	29	23
Soybean oil tub	45	35	20
Corn oil stick	59	24	17

[1] For butter, 11% of the monounsaturated fat is naturally occurring *trans*.

[2] About 50% of the saturated fat content of cocoa butter is stearic acid, which is not considered to be atherogenic.

[3] A portion of these fats are omega-3 fatty acids. Fatty fish such as mackerel, salmon (Pacific), tuna, herring, and trout contain the greatest quantities of omega-3 fatty acids.

[4] The average *trans*-fatty acid content of major brand stick and tub margarine is about 24% and 15% respectively.

[5] Notice that olive oil is highest in monounsaturated fats and canola oil is lowest in saturated fat. These two could be labeled the "most healthful fats."

ture. The monounsaturated fatty acid (**MUFA**) has one point of unsaturation. The polyunsaturated fatty acid (**PUFA**) has two or more points of unsaturation. The two essential fatty acids in the human diet are the **omega-6 (linoleic)** in leafy veggies, seeds, nuts, grains, oils and the **omega-3 (linolenic)** in oils, nuts, seeds (specifically flax), and soybeans.

Two other classes of lipids are **phospholipids**, which are similar to a triglyceride, but have a phosphorus-containing acid in place of one of the fatty acids (lecithin) and the **sterols**, which the most common is **cholesterol**, a soft waxy substance made by the liver and found in animal foods, but is not an essential nutrient. Although the body makes cholesterol and it is essential for cell membrane functioning, cholesterol is not needed in the diet, and too much can increase blood cholesterol levels and increase heart disease risk.

Dietary Fats

When comparing the fatty acid composition of different dietary fats, you will observe that canola oil has the lowest saturated fat, olive oil has the highest monounsaturated fat, and coconut oil is the highest in saturated fat. Because saturated fat has been linked to heart disease and studies have shown increased monounsaturated fats decrease heart disease, the recommendation is to eat more plant fats, specifically those with monounsaturated fats such as olive oil and avocado and tree nuts.

Processed and Damaged Fats

Although plant fats are generally healthful in their natural forms, processing and spoilage can turn them unhealthful. Hydrogenation is a process of adding hydrogen atoms under pressure that creates a trans fat that is different from any found in nature, but similar to a saturated fat. You should try to avoid hydrogenated and partially hydrogenated fats in foods because they increase blood cholesterol levels, decrease HDLs, and increase LDLs (explained in the "Metabolizing Fat" section). Check labels carefully (especially margarines). *Spectrum Naturals* has a healthful margarine that is nonhydrogenated and low in saturated fat. In order to minimize one's intake of trans fatty acids, one should not only limit the use of hydrogenated fats, but also limit deep-fried foods, high-fat baked goods, and the use of nondairy creamers.

In addition to processing, oils (especially polyunsaturated oils) are susceptible to decomposing when exposed to light. They will yield an unpleasant odor and flavor when rancid, and their shelf life is limited. To prevent rancidity and avoid hydrogenation, companies may add Vitamin E, BHA, and BHT. The consumer can help prevent rancidity by keeping the oil in a cool place away from direct sunlight and consuming it in a reasonable amount of time. Sometimes oils such as canola and safflower are refrigerated.

Digesting and Absorbing Fat

The digestion of fat involves the **liver** making bile, then the **gallbladder** storing it, and then releasing it into the small intestine. The bile emulsifies the fat. The **pancreas** releases an enzyme called **lipase** that splits triglycerides into monoglycerides, glycerol, and FA. Absorption of monoglycerides, glycerol, and FA occurs through the wall of the small intestine. Smaller fats are absorbed into the blood and carried as **lipoproteins**, and larger fats are absorbed into the lymphatic system as **chylomicrons**.

Metabolizing Fats

Once fats are absorbed, they are metabolized and transported by lipoprotein carriers. A **chylomicron** transports all the lipids as they enter the bloodstream. A very low density lipoprotein transports lipids made by the liver. A **high-density lipoprotein** that contains a large percentage of protein returns cholesterol from storage places to the liver for dismantling and disposal and thus is called the "good cholesterol." The **low-density lipoprotein** carrier contains a large percentage of cholesterol, transfers lipids from the liver to tissues, and has thus been called "bad cholesterol."

Fat Functions

Food fat and body fat serve many functions such as storing energy, cushioning vital organs, insulating the body and maintaining body temperature, transporting essential fatty acids and fat soluble vitamins, becoming part of cell membrane structure, offering satiety in meals, and enhancing food flavor and aroma.

Fat Needs

Although adult humans only need 3% of their Calories from linoleic acid and .3% of Calories from linolenic acid (a total of 3.3% Calories from essential fatty acids). The government recommendations are the following:

- **No more than 20–35% total fat, depending on the type of fats and personal health conditions**
- **< 65 grams/day for 2,000 kcal diet**
- **No more than 7–10% saturated fat**
- **Less than 300 mg from cholesterol**

The World Health Organization (WHO) recommends a lower limit of 0% for saturated fat, and progressive nutritionists such as Doctors McDougall, Ornish, and Pritikin suggest therapeutic recommendations of 10%–15%. A **20% total fat diet with 5%–6% maximum saturated fat and zero hydrogenated fat** is probably the most practical approach to fat consumption.

20% of Calories Fat Diet for Selected Daily Caloric Needs

Daily Caloric Intake	*Calories from Fat*	*Daily Fat Grams*
1400	280	31
1600	320	36
1800	360	40
2000	400	45
2200	440	49
2400	480	53
2600	520	58
2800	560	62
3000	600	67
3200	640	71
3400	680	76
3600	720	80
3800	760	84
4000	800	89
4200	840	93
4400	880	98
4600	920	102
4800	960	107
5000	1000	111

More on Essential Fatty Acids

Humans need essential fatty acids that the body cannot make for immune function, vision, cell membrane, and production of hormonelike compounds. One essential fatty acid needed, the omega-3 fatty acid called linolenic acid, is primarily from fish, canola, and soybean oil and also found in flax seeds and walnuts. Eicosapentaenoic acid (EPA) and docosahexaenoic acid (DHA) are made from these. It is recommended to eat fish 1–2 times per week or consume the plant sources given to also help decrease blood clot formation and lower your risk of heart disease. The omega-6 fatty acid, linoleic acid, is found in vegetable oils and helps to increase blood clot formation and increase inflammatory responses. Only 1 tablespoon a day is needed. Some signs and symptoms of essential fatty acid deficiency are flaky, itchy skin, diarrhea, infections, retarded growth and wound healing, and anemia.

Special Topic: Heart Disease

The special topic of the lipids chapter is heart disease because it is the number one killer of Americans. Plaque buildup can begin in childhood and take years to develop before one experiences a myocardial infarction or stroke from lack of blood flow through the arteries.

The following chart gives the risk factors associated with heart disease:

Conquering Heart Disease: Recognition of Risk Factors

Factor	***Female***	***Male***	***Children***
Age	> 55; younger women with multiple risk factors	> 50	N/A
Family history	First degree relative (parent or sibling) with premature heart attack (before age 55 in men and before 65 in women)		
Sex	Premature menopause without HRT	N/A	
Diabetes	Presence removes protective effects of estrogen	Diagnosis	
Hypertension	> 140 systolic > 90 diastolic. Elevated systolic alone (Isolated Systolic Hypertension) may also increase risk		N/A
Total cholesterol (mg/dL)	≥ 240 200–239 borderline		> 200
LDL cholesterol (mg/dL)	≥ 160 high 130–159 borderline		≥ 130 high 110–129 borderline
HDL cholesterol (mg/dL)	< 35		
Cholesterol/ HDL ratio	> 4.5	> 5.0	> 3.7
Triglycerides (mg/dL)	> 190 or > 150 with HDL < 40	N/A	
Body weight (BMI = kg/m^2)	BMI > 27.3 (NHS: BMI > 21; weight gain after 18 years of age)	BMI > 27.8; > 30% above ideal body weight	> 30% above ideal body weight
Waist/hip ratio	> 0.8	> 1.0	N/A
Physical inactivity	Yes		
Cigarette smoking	Yes		
Stress	Maybe	Yes	N/A

Comparison of Five Dietary Programs for Reducing Heart Attacks

Characteristics of Cholesterol-Lowering Diets

Dietary Component	***Recommended Intakes***				
	Step I	***Step II***[a]	***Pritikin***[b]	***Ornish***[c]	***AHA***[d]
Total fat	Less than 30% of calories		10% of total calories	10% of total calories	No RDA for fat
Saturated fats	< 10% of total calories	< 7% of total calories	Almost none	Almost none	8%–10% of TEI from saturated fat
Polyunsaturated fats	Up to 10% of total calories		Use caution	Half of fat intake	≤ 10% of TEI
Monounsaturated fats	10–15% of total calories		Use caution	Half of fat intake	≤ 15% of TEI
Cholesterol	< 300 mg/day	< 200 mg/day	< 100 mg	5 mg/day	≤ 300 mg
Carbohydrates	55% of total calories		75%–80%	70%–75%	
Protein	10–20% of total calories		10%–15%	15%–20%	
Total calories	To achieve and maintain desirable weight		At least 1,000 for women, 1,200 for men	No restriction	
Fiber	Increase soluble fiber to 15–25 g/day		> 35 g/day	Not specified	
Sodium	Not specified		< 1600 mg/day	Not specified	≤ 2400 mg

[a] The National Cholesterol Education Program's Step I and Step II diets.
[b] Pritikin Program
[c] Dean Ornish's Diet for Reversing Heart Disease
[d] AHA (American Heart Association) recommendations

Dietary Factors that May Increase Heart Disease Risk

Factor	***Proposed Mechanism***
Saturated fatty acids	Stimulate the liver to make more LDL cholesterol, decrease LDL receptors in liver.
Polyunsaturated fat	May decrease HDL, while decreasing LDL.
Trans-fatty acids	May increase LDL and may decrease HDL.
Dietary cholesterol	May have a minor effect when compared with intake of saturated fats. However, dietary cholesterol may raise serum cholesterol in some individuals.
Obesity	Elevated waist/hip ratio (android obesity) increases risk due to decreased HDLs. Obesity also increases risk for hypertension.
Homocysteine	Elevated levels may promote a greater buildup of arterial plaque and risk for severe thromboembolism. High levels often associated with low levels of vitamin B_6 and folic acid.
High sodium intake	Linked to hypertension in "salt-sensitive" individuals. Daily reference value is 2,500 mg/day.
Coffee oils (cafestol and kahweol)	Diterpenes increase total cholesterol. Problematic with French press and Turkish coffees. Coffee filters trap harmful oils, and drinking filtered coffee does not increase risk.
Iron	Promotes formation of free radicals, which can oxidize LDLs. However, Finnish study implicating iron as increasing risk for heart disease was not supported by recent U.S. studies.

The impact of your diet on your health is remarkable. The leading cause of death in the United States is heart disease. There are many associations between heart disease and diet. A few of these relationships are increased total fat in the diet, which increases one's chances of heart disease; increased saturated fat in one's diet, which may increase one's chances of heart disease; increased hydrogenated fats, which may increase one's chances of heart disease; increased phytochemicals, which may decrease one's chances of heart disease; and increased consumption of omega-3s and MUFA, which may decrease one's chances of heart disease. In summary, all lipids were not created equal.

 Dietary Factors that May Decrease Heart Disease Risk

Factor	Proposed Mechanism
Monounsaturated fats	♦ May reduce LDL cholesterol.
Garlic, onions	♦ Allicin and sulfide compounds may lower LDLs and raise HDLs.
Soybeans	♦ Soy protein lowers LDL cholesterol. ♦ Genistein inhibits smooth-muscle proliferation, plaque formation, and activity of thrombin. ♦ Soy milk may inhibit oxidation of LDL cholesterol.
Chromium	♦ Increased HDL in men with hypertension taking beta-blockers. Role in women unclear.
Water-soluble fiber	♦ Lowers cholesterol by altering absorption of bile salts. Gums and pectins (oats, oat bran, barley, legumes, prunes, apples, carrots and grapefruit), and mucilage (psyllium seeds) are examples.
Antioxidants	♦ Prevent oxidation of LDL cholesterol. Vitamin E (400 IU) most protective. Vitamin C, selenium, beta-carotene, phenolic compounds and melatonin may also be effective.
Alcohol	♦ Moderate consumption of 1–2 drinks per day (12 oz. beer, 5 oz. wine, or 1.5 oz 80 proof) may raise HDL levels. Hypertension linked with consumption of more than 3 drinks/day. ♦ Red wine (not white wine) contains phenolic compounds that act as antioxidants.
	♦ May break up blood clots by increasing tPA.
Melatonin	♦ May decrease LDLs and act as an antioxidant. ♦ Patients with heart disease had lower nighttime levels compared to controls.
Weight loss	♦ May lower triglycerides and blood pressure. Combined with exercise, weight loss may raise HDLs.
Potassium and calcium	♦ May decrease risk for hypertension; increase dietary potassium (citrus, bananas, dates, potato) and calcium (1,000–1,500 mg/day).
Omega-3 fatty acids	♦ Inhibit blood clotting and platelet aggregation.
Folic acid and Vitamin B_6	♦ Break down homocysteine; low levels increase risk.

 Quick Tip: Mediterranean Diets

◇ Diet is characterized by abundant plant foods (fruit, vegetables, breads, cereals, potatoes, beans, nuts, and seeds).

◇ Olive oil is the predominant source of fat. Because eggs, dairy products (principally cheese and yogurt), fish, and poultry are consumed in low to moderate amounts, and red meat is rarely consumed, the diet is low in saturated fat (< 7% of total calories).

◇ Wine is consumed in low to moderate amounts, normally with meals. Regular physical activity is encouraged.

chapter 6

Protein—Too Little or Too Much

Protein is one of the most important nutrients in the maintenance of good health and vitality. It is of vital importance in the growth and development of all body tissues. It provides a major source of building materials for blood, muscles, skin, hair, nails, and glands, as well as for hormones, enzymes, and antibodies. A diet deficient in protein may contribute to a variety of symptoms, yet most people in America get too much protein. The effects of too little and too much protein are discussed in this chapter, as well as the structure, digestion and absorption, functions, and requirements.

Protein Content of Selected Plant Foods

Food	Amount	Protein Grams
Tempeh	1 cup	31
Seitan	4 ounces	15–31
Soybeans, cooked	1 cup	29
Veggie dog	1 link	8–26
Veggie burger	1 patty	5–24
Lentils, cooked	1 cup	18
Tofu, firm	4 ounces	8–15
Kidney beans, cooked	1 cup	15
Lima beans, cooked	1 cup	15
Black beans, cooked	1 cup	15
Chickpeas, cooked	1 cup	15
Pinto beans, cooked	1 cup	14
Black-eyed peas, cooked	1 cup	13
Vegetarian baked beans	1 cup	12
Quinoa, cooked	1 cup	11
Soy milk, commercial, plain	1 cup	3–10
Tofu, regular	4 ounces	2–10
Bagel	1 medium (3 oz.)	9
Peas, cooked	1 cup	9
Textured vegetable protein, cooked	½ cup	8
Peanut butter	2 Tbsp.	8
Spaghetti, cooked	1 cup	7
Spinach, cooked	1 cup	6
Soy yogurt, plain	6 ounces	6
Bulgur, cooked	1 cup	6
Sunflower seeds	¼ cup	6
Almonds	¼ cup	6
Broccoli, cooked	1 cup	5
Whole wheat bread	2 slices	5
Cashews	¼ cup	5
Almond butter	2 Tbsp.	5
Brown rice, cooked	1 cup	5
Potato	1 medium (6 oz.)	4

Protein Content of Selected Animal-Derived Foods

Food	Amount	Protein Grams
Chicken, baked	3 oz.	28
Pork roast	3 oz.	25
Sirloin steak	3 oz.	24
Flounder, baked	3 oz.	21
Ground beef, lean, baked	3 oz.	20
Cow's milk	1 cup	8
Cheddar cheese	1 oz.	7
Egg	1 large	6
Cow milk yogurt	1 cup	8

Foods that are high in protein and high in fat are generally animal proteins, which are not essential in one's diet to meet protein needs. When choosing concentrated proteins for the diet, choose first beans and bean products, soy, peas, legumes, whole grains, potatoes, whole grains, and whole-grain cereals. Choose less often omega-3–rich fish then low-fat chicken and turkey. Choose the least pork, high-fat fish, dairy products, and eggs. Plant proteins do not need to be combined with other plant proteins in one meal to meet amino acid recommendations. A variety throughout the day is sufficient.

Protein Structures

There are 20 total **amino acids** in which 9 are essential. All amino acids have an amine group and an acid group, but vary in their structure by their varying side chains. Proteins are made up of strands of amino acids linked together by peptide bonds to form proteins. The strands coil and fold to make a variety of proteins for various functions. Eating a variety of foods from day to day will ensure that all amino acid needs are met in the diet.

Digesting and Absorbing Proteins

Protein digestion starts with the stomach acids denaturing protein and the stomach enzyme pepsin starting to split the protein chains. The pancreas releases the enzyme **trypsin,** and the small intestine releases enzymes that further break apart proteins into **tripeptides**, then **dipeptides**, and then individual amino acids. Absorption of the amino acids occurs through the wall of the small intestine into the bloodstream, and they are carried to the liver, then to the rest of the body.

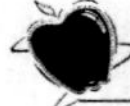

Essential and Nonessential Amino Acids

Essential (indispensable) amino acids	Nonessential (dispensable) amino acids
Histidine	Alanine
Isoleucine	Arginine
Leucine	Asparagine
Lysine	Aspartic acid
Methionine	Cysteine
Phenylalanine	Cystine
Threonine	Glutamic acid
Tryptophan	Glutamine
Valine	Glycine
	Proline
	Serine
	Tyrosine

Protein Functions

The primary functions of protein are the following:

- **Growth and maintenance of tissue**
- **Enzyme and hormone development**
- **Making antibodies (to fight infection)**
- **Fluid and electrolyte balance (too much can cause dehydrated cells)**
- **Acid-base balance, and**
- **Energy (as a last resort) by a process called gluconeogenesis.**

Protein and Malnutrition

Protein deficiencies around the world have been linked to malnutrition. There are three general types of malnutrition: protein-energy malnutrition, kwashiorkor, and marasmus. Protein-energy malnutrition is a form of malnutrition in which lack of protein is directly related to a lack of Calories in starving areas of the world. Kwashiorkor is a disease from a low-protein-dense diet where energy needs are marginally met. Some signs and symptoms are apathy, listlessness, failure to grow, poor weight gain, change in hair color, nutrient deficiency, flaky skin, fatty infiltration in the liver, and massive edema in the abdomen and legs. Some characteristics of marasmus are starving to death, insufficient protein, insufficient energy, insufficient nutrients, "skin and bones" appearance, little or no subcutaneous fat, and reduced brain growth.

Balancing Protein Needs with Intake

Protein requirements and recommendations are based on many years of scientific research. Charts are established from these studies based on body weight, sex, and age. Athletes do not generally need extra protein unless they are trying to gain muscle mass or they engage in endurance sports. The DRI for protein for most people is .8 grams per kilogram of body weight, and it is 1–1.5 grams per kilogram of body weight for endurance athletes and bodybuilders. It is important to notice that the calculations are based on body weight in kilograms, not in pounds. Additional recommendations include increasing plant proteins and keeping the percentage to 10%–15% of total Calories for any person who is within their appropriate caloric range. The following is a chart of estimated protein needs of various populations.

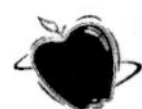

Population	***Estimated protein needs per day***
Adult male (25–50 years)	63 grams
Adult female (25–50 years)	50 grams
Pregnant female	60–75 grams
Child (7–10 years)	28 grams
Endurance athlete and bodybuilder	Generally 1.2 grams per kilogram of body weight
Vegan	Same as one's age/sex group

The following is an example of how you would calculate your personal protein needs.

0.8 gm of protein/kg of healthy body weight

$$\frac{140\text{ lb.}}{2.2\text{ kg/lb.}} = 64\text{ kg}$$

$$64\text{ kg} \times \frac{0.8\text{ g protein}}{\text{kg healthy body wt}} = 51\text{ g protein}$$

Protein Requirements Based on Weight for the Average Adult Person

Body Weight	Protein Intake in Grams
100	36
110	40
120	44
130	47
140	51
150	55
160	58
170	62
180	65
200	73
220	80
230	84
240	87
250	91

The following chart shows the **protein grams** for selected percentages of protein.

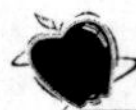

% of Calories Fat	1500 Calorie	2000 Calorie	2500 Calorie	3000 Calorie	3500 Calorie	4000 Calorie
5%	19	25	31	38	38	50
10%	38	50	63	**75**	88	100
15%	56	75	94	113	131	150
20%	75	100	125	150	175	200
25%	94	125	156	188	219	250
30%	113	150	187	225	263	300

When you consider that .8 grams per kilogram of body weight meets your protein needs and plug that number into the chart, you will find that **10%–15%** is an appropriate recommendation for each caloric level. Exceptions to the 10%–15% recommendation may be for a recovering anorexic that may need a higher percentage because of the deficient Calories and athletes that may need a lower **percentage** (although higher grams) to meet their needs because of their abundance of Calories for meeting energy needs.

For the following example, an 18-year-old male weighs 170 pounds.

0.8 gm of protein/kg of healthy body weight

$$\frac{170\text{ lb.}}{2.2\text{ kg/lb.}} = 77\text{ kg}$$

$$77\text{ kg} \times \frac{0.8\text{ g protein}}{\text{kg healthy body wt}} = 62\text{ g protein}$$

Because the recommended energy intake for an 18-year-old male is 3000 Calories daily, look at the 3000 Calorie column and find that 62 grams of protein is less than 75 grams of protein, so this individual would actually need slightly less than 10% of Calories from protein. Notice that recommending a 30% fat diet (as in the Zone diet) will give this male example 225 grams of protein for the day (3.6 times his needs and a burden to his body)!

Too Much Protein

It is difficult to not get enough protein if you eat an appropriate amount of Calories for your body weight. There are dangers of overdosing on two times or more the recommended amount of protein. Dangers are **weight gain** if too many Calories are eaten, **water loss** (dehydration) if carbohydrates are not consumed, excess **calcium excretion** (which can lead to osteoporosis), and possible **kidney problems**. High animal protein in the diet increases the risk of heart disease and colon cancer. The National Academy of Sciences recommends consuming no more than two times one's individual RDA for protein in a day. In summary, protein is essential and vital for our body's functioning, but Americans suffer from excess protein illness more often than protein deficiency.

chapter 7

Vegetarian Nutrition—Facts, Myths, and More!

Vegetarian diets are common around the world, and an understanding of this lifestyle choice will not only help those who want to consume a more plant-based diet, but also shed light on the myths associated with vegetarianism and help nonvegetarians to be not only tolerant, but also more accepting of those whose cultures or beliefs include vegetarian diets.

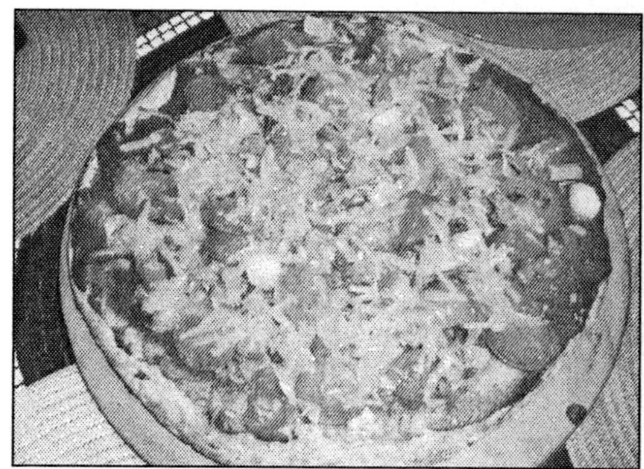
Vegan Pizza

Types of Vegetarians

Vegetarian diets are those that do not include eating the flesh of an animal that has died (sometimes stated as anything that had a face). Vegetarians eat plant diets of grains, legumes, nuts, seeds, soy products, vegetables, fruits, oils, and sweets. A **lacto-ovo vegetarian** also eats dairy products and eggs. A **lacto vegetarian** includes the dairy, but not the eggs. An **ovo-vegetarian** includes the eggs, although no dairy. There are many food guide plans for vegetarians, but vegetarians may use the USDA pyramid by just eliminating the animal flesh foods from the protein category. As shown in chapter 2, Oldways developed a pyramid that reflects healthful vegetarian diets around the world. The Healthful House also emphasizes plant food over animal foods.

Vegans are vegetarians that include all those foods listed previously for vegetarians, excluding the dairy and eggs. Some subgroups of vegetarian and vegan diets are fruitarian and raw food diets that include primarily nuts, seeds, and fruits and the macrobiotic diets that include generally brown rice, some veggies, and soy products. An example of a vegan's diet on one day may be:

Breakfast—Whole-grain waffles with almond butter and pure maple syrup topped with blueberries, strawberries, and papaya and a glass of soy milk or calcium-fortified grapefruit juice.

Lunch—Baked tofu sandwich on a whole-grain bun with tomato, avocado, lettuce, and mustard, peach soy yogurt with ground flax and walnut sprinkles, and carrot sticks with hummus.

Dinner—Homemade pesto pasta (pesto from basil, pine nuts, garlic, and olive oil) with green beans and tomatoes sprinkled with soy parmesan, seven-color garden salad with balsamic-vinaigrette dressing and fresh nine-grain bread with spectrum naturals non-hydrogenated margarine.

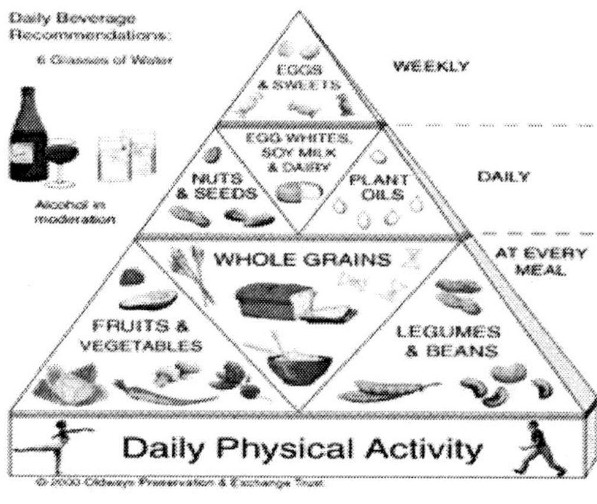

© 2000 Oldways Preservation & Exchange Trust, http://oldwayspt.org

Reasons for Being Vegetarian

People from various cultural backgrounds all over the world choose to be vegetarians for many different reasons. Some of those reasons are ethical or religious (Buddhism, Hinduism, Seventh Day Adventists, and Essenes), some are for more personal, athletic, or health reasons (reducing chances

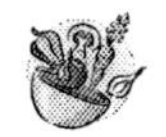

Types of Vegetarians:

Lacto-ovo:	Eats dairy and eggs in addition to plant foods
Lacto:	Eats dairy in addition to plant foods
Ovo:	Eats eggs in addition to plant foods
Vegan:	Eats no animal products; eats legumes, whole grains, veggies, fruits, and products from these sources

of heart disease, cancer, stroke, obesity, and diabetes), and some are more global reasons such as to make a lifestyle choice to help the environment and feed the world more economically and resourcefully, conserving water, land, and rain forests.

Perceived Nutritional Concerns

Often when the topic of vegetarianism comes up, nutrient concerns are raised. Many of those concerns are actually myths because vegetarians can meet nutrient needs as easily as nonvegetarians, if not even more readily because of the conscious decision to eat a more healthful diet. For instance, it is very easy to get enough protein from veggies, nuts, grains, and beans. **Iron** is available in prunes, dried fruit, blackstrap molasses, peas, tofu, tomato juice, butternut squash, brussels sprouts, dark greens, beans, and fortified foods. Vitamin C foods such as dark greens also contain iron that is highly absorbable with the vitamin C. **Calcium** is also easily attainable in a variety of foods such as kale, mustard greens, turnip greens, bok choy, sea veggies, broccoli, blackstrap molasses, legumes, dried figs, fortified OJ, tofu, corn tortillas, fortified soy, and rice milk. Calcium needs are actually less on a lower (but adequate) protein diet. The best sources of calcium come from where the cows get it—dark greens. Equal in calcium and vitamin D to cow's milk is soy and brown rice milk. Of course one's own mother's milk is the best source of calcium (as well as other nutrients) and is the optimal milk beverage of choice for infants and toddlers. **B_{12}** is one nutrient that comes from bacteria in animals (like us), but vegan sources such as nutritional yeast, fortified cereals, fortified soy milks, and soy products can meet one's needs. Whether nutrient needs are met is not dependent on whether a person is vegetarian or not vegetarian, but whether someone is choosing nutrient-dense foods. Also, many silly myths have been said of vegetarians that are not true such as vegetarians are hippies, vegetarians can only be women, vegetarians are wimps, vegetarians cannot eat out, and vegetarians have to spend a lot of time planning and cooking meals.

Sample Menu Showing How Easy It Is to Meet Protein Needs with Plant Foods

	Protein (gms)
Breakfast:	
1 cup oatmeal	6
1 cup soymilk	9
1 bagel	9
Lunch:	
2 slices whole wheat bread	5
1 cup Vegetarian Baked Beans	12
Dinner:	
5 oz. firm tofu	16
1 cup cooked broccoli	5
1 cup cooked brown rice	5
2 Tbsp. almonds	3
Snack:	
2 Tbsp. peanut butter	8
6 crackers	2
TOTAL	80 grams

Protein Recommendations for Male Vegan, 63–79 grams
[based on 0.8–1 gram of protein per kilogram body weight for 79-kilogram (174-pound) male]

Comparing a Vegetarian Diet to an Animal-Based Diet

When comparing a vegetarian diet to a meat-based diet, the vegetarian diet usually has more fiber and complex carbs, less fat, less but adequate protein, less food-borne illness, more phytochemicals, less cholesterol, and less saturated fat. Some benefits of vegetarian diets then are generally less overfat problems, less heart disease, less chance of diabetes and better control of it, less GI and colon problems, less cancers, and less osteoporosis. Dr. Dean Ornish, Dr. John McDougall, and Dr. Michael Klaper all put patients on a vegetarian or near vegetarian diet for its healing effects on these diseases.

More Details About Plant-Based Proteins

Tempeh (TEM-pay) is an Indonesian main staple consisting of soybeans, grain, and a rice culture. Tempeh makes for a sweet delicate meat that can be charbroiled, sauteed, or fried.

Nutritional Information

- A complete protein, contains all eight amino acids
- Vegetarian source of vitamin B_{12}
- High in iron
- Zero cholesterol
- High in fiber and soluble fiber, which is cholesterol reducing

Seitan (SAY-tahn) wheat meat! Seitan is 100% wheat protein or gluten. Historically seitan has been utilized for over 2,000 years in China and the Near East. Seitan is made by kneading wheat flour, then rinsing with water until starch is removed and the pure protein (gluten) is retained.

Nutritional Information

- A complete protein source
- Zero fat content
- No cholesterol
- Half the calories of beef

Soy protein is made from defatted soy flour, which is then cooked under pressure and dried. Soy protein can be hydrated and added to many delicious recipes.

Nutritional Information Per ¼-cup Serving (dry)

- Zero cholesterol
- 7 grams protein
- .1 gram fat
- 4 grams carbohydrates

Eating a More Plant-Based Diet

An excellent web site to check out for vegetarian diets is http://www.vrg.org/ for the Vegetarian Resource Group. Some popular magazines are *Vegetarian Times* and *Vegetarian Journal.* Plan your meals around starches and seasonal veggies and try eating more international meals. Anyone can benefit from learning to add more phytonutrient and antioxidant-rich foods to the diet. Learning to include more plant-based foods or consuming an entirely vegetarian diet can be a lifestyle full of advantages and rewards.

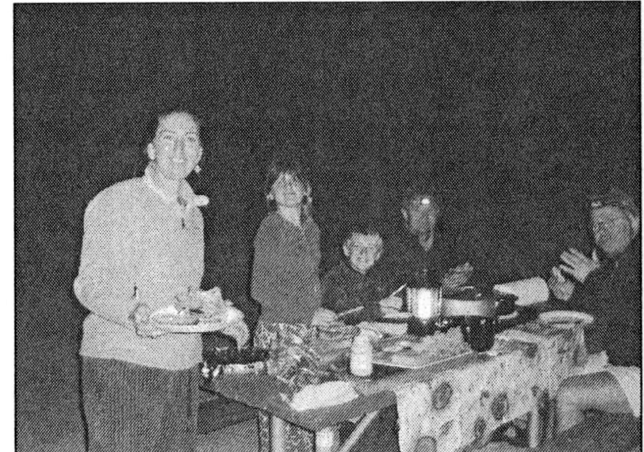

Families Love Veggie Burgers while Camping!

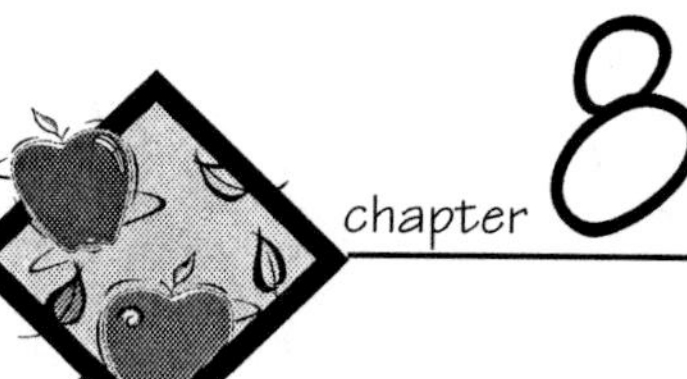

Vitamins, Minerals, and Phytochemicals for Health and Sport

There are about 13 vitamins and 21 minerals that are essential for health. Although neither of these provides Calories (energy) for the body, they are critical metabolizing nutrients that the body needs in order to function. Vitamins, which are organic, generally facilitate energy-yielding chemical reactions and can be categorized into fat-soluble (**ADEK**) and water soluble (**C and the Bs**). Fat-soluble vitamins dissolve in organic solvents and are not readily excreted, so they may cause toxicity in the body. They must be absorbed with fat and transported with fat in the body. The water-soluble vitamins dissolve in water, generally are readily excreted, function as coenzymes, and are subject to cooking losses. Minerals are also non-energy-yielding nutrients that have various functions in the body and can be categorized into major (**Ca, P, Mg, Na, K, Cl, and S**) and trace (including **Fe, Zn, Se, Cr, I, F, and Cu**). The major minerals are those humans need more than 100 grams a day. Trace minerals are those that humans need less than 100 milligrams a day. The following charts list each vitamin and mineral in these categories and list their functions, deficiency diseases and symptoms, toxicity problems, and healthful food sources. Some rich food sources have been left out if they contain excessive amounts of saturated fat or cholesterol.

The Fat-Soluble Vitamins

Nutrient	Vitamin A	Vitamin D	Vitamin E	Vitamin K
Function	Vision	Bone mineralization	RBC formation and prevents RBC damage	Blood clotting
	Linings	Maintains blood calcium levels	Antioxidant	
	Acts as an antioxidant	Transports calcium to muscles	Promotes aerobic energy production	
Deficiency Diseases and Symptoms	Night blindness	Rickets—children (bowed legs)	Fibrocystic breast disease	
	Xerophthalmia	Osteomalacia in adults (softening of bones)	Rupture of RBC	
	Hypovitaminosis A			
	Stunted growth			
	Impaired immunity			
Toxicity Problems	Birth defects over 10,000 IU	Most toxic vitamin (At only 4–5 x RDA)	Bleeding (rare)	Breaking of RBC
	Enlarged liver/spleen Sore muscles	Headache		Interferes with anticoagulants
	Hair loss	Nausea		Brain damage
		Calcium deposit in tissues		
Healthful Food Sources	Beta carotene: Dark and leafy greens, broccoli, deep orange veggies and fruits (carrots, sweet potatoes, apricots, pumpkin)	Sunshine causes body to synthesis	Nuts, seeds, vegetable oils and margarine, wheat germ, whole grains, dark green leafy veggies	Synthesized by intestinal bacteria
	Retinol: Fortified cow's milk and soy milk, cheese and eggs	Fortified soy, cow's, and brown rice milk		Dark leafy green vegetables

The Water-Soluble Vitamins

Nutrient	*Vitamin B_1 (Thiamin)*	*Vitamin B_2 (Riboflavin)*	*Vitamin B_3 (Niacin)*	*Vitamin B_6 (Pyridoxine)*
Function	Acts as a coenzyme in metabolism of energy nutrients (C, F, P) Formation of hemoglobin Proper nervous system functioning	Metabolism of energy nutrients (C, F, P) Vision and healthy skin	Metabolism of energy nutrients (C, F, P) Treatment for high cholesterol and artery blockage	Metabolism of amino acids Formation of hemoglobin and oxidative enzymes Proper nervous system functioning
Deficiency Diseases and Symptoms	Beri-beri Paralysis of legs Mental confusion	Ariboflavinosis (cracks in the corner of the mouth)	Pellagra Dermatitis Diarrhea	Antimetabolites: Alcohol Birth control pills Weakens immunity
Toxicity Problems	No symptoms reported	No symptoms reported	Face flushes (red) at 10 x RDA Liver toxicity	Over 2 grams daily (PMS patients using)
Healthful Food Sources	Whole grains, wheat germ, legumes, nuts	Whole grains, dairy, dark green leafy veggies, enriched grains	Whole grains, nuts, enriched grains, fish, poultry	Need is proportional to protein intake Legumes, green and leafy veggies, whole grains, potatoes, fish, poultry

Nutrient	*Vitamin B_{12}*	*Folate*	*Pantothenic Acid*	*Vitamin C*
Function	RBC and other cell formation (coenzyme) Nervous system function	Coenzyme used in synthesis of new cells (i.e., RBC)	Coenzyme in energy metabolism	Maintain collagen and connective tissue Antioxidant Immunity Increases absorption of iron Promotion of aerobic energy production
Deficiency Diseases and Symptoms	Pernicious anemia caused by lack of intrinsic factor Nerve damage and paralysis Megaloblastic anemia	Megoloblastic anemia Neural tube birth defects (i.e., spina bifida) Depression	Rare Vomiting	Scurvy Bleeding gums Failure of wounds to heal Depleted during stress
Toxicity Problems	None reported	May mask B_{12} deficiency	None reported at 10–20 gm/day	Diarrhea, nausea, gas Possible hardening of the arteries
Healthful Food Sources	Fortified soy milk, nutritional yeast, meat analogs, fortified cereals, (all animal foods have B_{12} because it is synthesized by the intestines)	Leafy green vegetables, legumes (lentils the highest), seeds, orange juice	Widespread in whole foods like whole grains and legumes	Citrus fruits (orange, strawberry, grapefruit, tomatoes), dark greens, potatoes, peppers, cantaloupe

The Major Minerals

Nutrient	Calcium (Ca)	Phosphorus (P)	Magnesium (Mg)
Function	Bones and teeth Muscle contraction/relaxation Normal blood pressure Immune defenses Blood clotting Glycogen breakdown	Bones and teeth Genetic material in cell Phospholipids in cell membranes Energy Transfer (formation of ATP/CP) Buffering systems Release of O_2 from RBC	Bone mineralization Muscle contraction Building of protein Enzyme action Nerve transmission Teeth maintenance Glucose metabolism in muscle cell
Deficiency Diseases and Symptoms	Children: stunted growth Adults: bone loss (osteoporosis) Excess protein and phosphorus may deplete	Bone pain Impaired growth Rickets in infants	Children: growth failure Weakness Confusion, convulsions, hallucinations
Toxicity Problems	Excess excreted	Excretes calcium	Confusion Lack of muscle coordination Coma or death
Healthful Food Sources	Legumes, greens, nonfat dairy, enriched soy and rice milk, Ca-fortified orange juice	Most whole foods (legumes, whole grains, fish, nuts)	Whole grains, legumes, greens, nuts, seafood, chocolate

Nutrient	Sodium (Na)	Potassium (K)	Chloride (Cl)	Sulfur (S)
Function	Fluid and electrolyte balance Maintains acid-base balance in cell Nerve impulse transmission Muscle contraction Form table salt with chloride	Fluid and electrolyte balance Nerve impulse transmission Muscle contraction (including heart) Glycogen storage Protein synthesis	Part of HCL in stomach Fluid balance Acid-base balance	Component of: Some amino acids Biotin Thiamin Insulin Stabilizes protein shape Detoxifies harmful compounds
Deficiency Diseases and Symptoms	Muscle cramps Apathy Caused from excessive sweating in endurance exercise	Dehydration Weakness Paralysis caused from excessive sweating, laxatives, diarrhea, or vomiting	Muscle cramps Apathy Growth failure in children	None known
Toxicity Problems	Hypertension (high blood pressure)	Muscular weakness Vomiting, can stop heart if given into vein	Normally harmless (gas is poisonous)	Occurs only if sulfur amino acids eaten in excess—depresses growth
Healthful Food Sources	Enough in whole foods (excess from salt, soy sauce, processed foods, fast food)	All whole foods (especially fruits and vegetables)	Enough in whole foods (excess from salt, processed foods, fast food, soy sauce)	All protein-containing foods

The Trace Minerals

Nutrient	***Iron (Fe)***	***Zinc (Zn)***	***Selenium (Se)***
Function	Part of hemoglobin in blood Part of myoglobin in muscles O_2 transport O_2 for muscle contraction Immunity	Energy production in muscle Part of insulin and enzymes Immunity Taste perception Wound healing Makes genetic material Makes sperm	Antioxidant mineral Works with vitamin E
Deficiency Diseases and Symptoms	Anemia Weakness Lowered cold tolerance Infection	Growth failure in children Loss of taste Sexual retardation Wound healing	Sperm decreased Muscle degeneration Heart damage Fragile RBC
Toxicity Problems	Liver injury, infections, heart disease in some men, growth retardation in children	Fe absorption Anemia Artherosclerosis Kidney failure Diarrhea Vomiting	Muscle damage Hair and nail changes Liver damage
Healthful Food Sources	Legumes, dried fruits, greens, lean meats, tofu, fortified cereals, whole grains, cast iron cookware Vitamin C absorption	Whole grains, vegetables and protein-containing foods	Grains and veggies grown on Se-rich soil, seafood

Nutrient	***Chromium (Cr)***	***Iodine (I)***	***Fluoride (F)***	***Copper (Cu)***
Function	Help control blood glucose and insulin levels Needed for energy release of glucose	Component of thyroxine (thyroid hormone) Regulates growth and metabolism	Helps form bones and teeth (not essential to ingest) Helps teeth resist decay	Helps form hemoglobin Part of enzymes Close work w/Fe O_2 transport and utilization
Deficiency Diseases and Symptoms	Abnormal blood glucose metabolism	Goiter, cretinism	Tooth decay	Anemia Poor wound healing
Toxicity Problems	Possible muscle degeneration from supplementation	Depressed thyroid Goiter-like thyroid enlargement	Fluorosis (staining of teeth), chest pain, itching, nausea, vomiting	Vomiting Diarrhea
Healthful Food Sources	Whole grains, vegetable oils, lean meats	Iodized salt, seafood, bread, most plants	Fluoridated drinking water, toothpaste, supplements, sea products	Legumes, whole grains, nuts, dried fruit, drinking water

Phytochemicals have been in the forefront of recent nutrition research as new ones are being discovered. Phytochemicals are plant chemicals that have no nutritional value, but seem to be influential in many of the body's metabolic processes. Antioxidants and phytochemicals specifically benefit the health by the following.

- Suppressing DNA and protein synthesis
- Altering cell membrane structure and integrity
- Detoxifying carcinogenic compounds
- Affecting enzyme activity
- Preventing formation of excess oxygen-free radicals (i.e., vitamin E may block oxidation of serum cholesterol)
- Blocking cell receptors for natural hormones (i.e., phytoestrogens may suppress cancer developments this way)

Consumption of phytochemicals and antioxidants (collectively called nutraceuticals) from the whole plant themselves is recommended as health professionals believe there may be a collective effect of the various compounds in each food. Two books, *The Color Code: A Revolutionary Eating Plan for Optimal Health* by Joseph and Nadeau and *What Color is Your Diet?* by Heber, explain the various phytonutrients as categorized by color codes. The following is a summary of the color code research and possible health effect:

- Red: Tomatoes, tomato products, and watermelon contain lycopene, which may help males to prevent prostate cancer.
- Orange: Carrots and melon contain carotenoids, which may reduce risk of heart disease.
- Yellow: Yellow squash (dark yellow foods fight certain eye diseases).
- Green: Broccoli and kale contain sulforaphane, which may help prevent cancer.
- Blue-Purple: Blueberries and eggplant contain anthocyanins, which may help lower your blood pressure.
- White: Onion and garlic contain allicin, which may help lower cholesterol.

Remember the colors of the rainbow (ROY G. BIV) and choose one per group per day, as recommended in the Healthful House of Food and Fitness.

The following chart lists additional specific possible disease-fighting properties of selected phytochemicals with specific food sources.

Phytochemicals in Food and Their Possible Health Effects

Active Food Component	Possible Disease-Fighting Properties	Food Sources
Allylic sulfides	Inhibits cholesterol synthesis and protects against carcinogens	Garlic
Alpha-linolenic acid	Reduces inflammation and stimulates the immune system	Flax seed, soy products, walnuts
Capsaicin	Modulates blood clotting	Hot peppers
Carotenoids	Antioxidants that may protect against cancer and heart disease	Deeply pigmented fruits and veggies (carrots, winter squash, sweet potatoes, yams, cantaloupe, apricots, spinach, kale, citrus fruits, turnip greens, parsley, broccoli, pumpkin, tomatoes)
Catechins	May aid immune system and lower cholesterol	Green tea and berries
Coumarins	Prevents blood clotting and may have anticancer activity	Parsley, citrus fruits, carrots
Curcumin	May inhibit enzymes that activate carcinogens	Tumeric
Flavinoids	Act as antioxidants, scavenges carcinogens, binds to nitrites in the stomach, and prevents conversion to nitrosamines	Parsley, carrots, citrus fruits, broccoli, cabbage, cucumbers, squash, yams, tomatoes, eggplant, peppers, soy products, berries, black tea, celery, olives, onions, green tea, whole wheat, purple grapes, oregano, wine
Gamma-glutamyl allylic cysteines	May help lower blood pressure and elevate immune system activities	Garlic
Indoles	May inhibit estrogen action and triggers the production of enzymes that block DNA damage from carcinogens	Cruciferous veggies (broccoli, brussels sprouts, cabbage, cauliflower, kale) and horseradish and mustard greens
Isothiniocyanates	Inhibits enzymes that activate carcinogens and triggers production of enzymes that detoxify carcinogens	Same foods as "indoles"
Liminoids	Induces protective enzymes	Citrus fruits
Lignins	Blocks estrogen activity in cells, possibly reducing the risk of cancer of the breast, colon, prostate, and ovaries	Flax seed and its oils, whole grains
Lycopene	Antioxidant that helps the body resist cancer and its progression	Tomatoes and red grapefruit
Monoterpenes	Antioxidant that inhibits cholesterol production and aids in protective enzyme activity	Citrus fruit peels, oils, parsley, carrots, broccoli, cabbage, cucumbers, squash, yams, tomatoes, eggplant, peppers, mint
Organosulfur Compounds	May speed production of carcinogen-destroying enzymes and may slow production of carcinogen-activating enzymes	Garlic, leeks, onions, chives
Phenolic acids	May help the body to resist cancer by inhibiting nitrosamine formation and affecting enzyme activity	Parsley, carrots, broccoli, cabbage, tomatoes, eggplant, peppers, citrus fruits, whole grains, berries, soybeans, oats, potatoes, coffee beans, apples, grapes, pears, prunes, and blueberries
Phytic acid	Binds to minerals, preventing free-radical formation, possibly reducing cancer risk	Whole grains

(continued)

Phytochemicals in Food and Their Possible Health Effects *(continued)*

Active Food Component	Possible Disease-Fighting Properties	Food Sources
Phthalides	Stimulates production of beneficial enzymes that detoxify carcinogens	Parsley, carrots, celery
Phytosterols (genestein and diadzin)	Estrogen inhibition may inhibit cell replication in GI tract, reduce risk of breast, colon, ovarian, prostate, and other estrogen-sensitive cancers and reduce cell survival and reduce risk of osteoporosis	Soybeans, soy flour, soy milk, tofu, textured vegetable protein, and other legume products
Protease inhibitors	May suppress enzyme activity in cancer cells, slowing tumor growth and inhibiting malignant changes in cells	All soy products, potatoes, and broccoli sprouts
Saponins	May interfere with DNA replication, preventing cancer cells from multiplying and may stimulate the immune response	Sprouts, potatoes, tomatoes, and green veggies
Tannins	An antioxidant that may inhibit carcinogen activation and cancer promotion	Black-eyed peas, lentils, grapes, red and white wine, tea
Triterpenoids	Prevents dental decay and acts as an antiulcer agent. Binds to estrogen and inhibits cancer by suppressing unwanted enzyme activity	Citrus fruits, licorice-root extract, soy products

chapter 9

Nutrition for Fat Loss and Weight Maintenance

Body Weight and Composition and Determining Ideals

Weight has become one of the most common obsessions of the American people. Weight loss books, videos, food, cremes, centers, and other gimmicks are a multi-billion dollar industry that continues to grow with the latest fads being diets that restrict the very nutrient that athletes and active people need the most of—carbohydrates!

Who determines how much you should weigh? The popular standard Metropolitan height-weight tables have been used to give people a range of ideal weight for their given height and have been revised over the years. Currently **BMI (Body Mass Index)** values are often used to determine overfatness or obesity. The formula to calculate your BMI is your weight in kilograms divided by your height squared in meters. Charts have been established to locate your BMI more quickly without calculating the formula. Unfortunately, each of these only use height and weight in the determination of body weight. These methods of assessments and many methods of weight loss fail to recognize the most important determinant of fat loss and positive body fitness changes—body composition testing.

The composition of the body is how much of the body is fat, how much is lean tissue or fat-free weight (muscle, bone, organs, etc.), and how much is water. The average person has between 55–60% of their total body weight composed of water. For example, a 150-pound may carry about 90 pounds of body water. Therefore, any quick changes in weight are a result in water loss and water gain. Most 5–10-pound fluctuations on the scale (especially for women pre-menstruation) are the result of water loss and gain. Scale poundage lost during exercise is a result of water loss. Throw out the weight scales—they are doing no good in telling you how your fat loss program is progressing. The only use for scales is for athletes to recognize how much to replenish fluid losses by drinking 2 cups of water for every pound of weight lost. As a matter of fact, most athletes that are eating a diet plentiful in carbohydrates such as fruits, vegetables and whole grains will increase their body water because for every gram of glycogen, 3 grams of water are retained. High-protein diets do the opposite—they dehydrate the cells and cause the body to retain fewer fluids. Sometimes, when you begin exercising you will gain total weight and lose fat because you will gain more body water, blood volume, and lean body tissue than you lose in fat so the net balance is a gain in weight, but a lower body fat percentage. In short, to adequately measure your fat loss from your new lifestyle changes (exercise and healthier eating) then you need to dump the scale and see how you look and feel and get your body composition estimated.

Body Composition can be estimated by several techniques now—the gold standard being underwater weighing in a tank. Other methods are skinfold measurements taken from a skilled technician, electric impedance, infrared, and the "bod pod." The accuracy of these techniques varies with factors such as technicians, time of day, and water retention, but the best guideline is that whatever you choose, go back to the same person and same type of test the next time for a useful comparison.

Body Composition for Optimal Health and Athletic Performance

Obviously, overfatness is a disadvantage in many sports such as running, cycling, soccer, and basketball. Optimal body fat percentages vary for each sport and each individual. Obesity is hazardous to your health by increasing your chances of many diseases including heart disease, diabetes, and hypertension. Although there are biological and genetic factors predisposing some people to obesity, lifestyle habits and choices have the greatest impact on your body composition. Even the maternal lifestyle choice of breast feeding greatly reduces a child's chances of childhood obesity and overfatness. Underactivity, food choices, and eating disorders are the main lifestyle choices that influence weight. Understanding the balance between energy nutrients, calories, and your exercise program are key to achieving an optimal body fat percentage that is right for you.

Fad Diets

When you know the basics about nutrition, it becomes easier to recognize fad diets and evaluate the positives and negatives of them. It also becomes apparent why some people feel they work. One of the most important basics in nutrition is that **one pound of fat is equal to 3500 Calories**. It is only possible to burn an extra 3500 Calories in one day by doing long intense exercise for several hours. Any weight loss program that claims to burn more than 1–2 pounds per week is promoting the loss of water weight, which is so easily gained back. The chart on page 65 gives the details of a few fad diets.

Summary of the High-Protein and High-Fat Diets

Many people lose weight when they begin a low-carbohydrate diet because of the body water loss. It does not matter how much water you drink. When carbs are stored as glycogen, they package more water along with them. In addition, excess protein will disrupt the body's fluid/electrolyte balance by excreting more water in the process of deamination (getting rid of excess nitrogen from the protein that needs to be used for energy because the person did not eat enough carbs). Some people are losing weight simply because they are on a low-calorie diet (under 2000 calories a day). Any diet low in calories will promote initial weight loss, but may also slow your metabolism, which is exactly what you do not want to do in a fat loss program.

Along with possible kidney, liver, and heart problems and osteoporosis, the low-carb diets are detrimental to an athlete's performance. Low glycogen stores are always a disadvantage for an athlete. An endurance athlete will need 500–700 grams of carbohydrates a day preceding competition (see Chapter 16) in order to have the glycogen storage to allow fat burning to occur during the competition. Even in ultraendurance events, the body burns 40–50% of its calories from carbs. The only athletes that are succeeding on the low percentage of carbs are the ones that are eating so many calories that they still receive the grams they need. Many women triathletes have bonked and crawled across finish lines that have not adhered to the proper carb storage guidelines. Athletes can train their muscles to almost double their carb storage and are burning carbs throughout the day so it is easy for a conditioned athlete to need 700–800 grams of carb storage in the muscles preceding competition.

Most of the low-carb programs classify all carbs as the same (see Chapter 4). Athletes need to eat diets rich in the unrefined complex carbohydrates such as fresh vegetables, brown rice, legumes, and whole grains such as kamut and oats. The list is quite long of nutritious carbohydrate foods, but unfortunately many Americans only know doughnuts and coffeecake so it is no wonder that carbs have been causing people problems. It is not the carbs that need to leave, but the sugary breakfast cereals (over 1/4 sugars) and coffee with sugary muffin!

The glycemic index that is discussed in many of the low-carb diets implies that even whole foods (i.e., bananas, raisins, carrots, corn, potatoes, pineapple, and watermelon) that have been found to cause a high sugar reaction in your body should always be avoided. Unfortunately, the books fail to

Popular Fad Diets and Their Effects

Diet Program	Premise	Author's Background	Calorie and Energy Nutrient Recommendations	Negative Health Implications	Validity
The Zone	Rigid obscure rules for eating	Barry Sears has a Ph.D. in biochemistry and no formal training in nutrition.	800–1200 Calories 40% carb 30% protein 30% fat	Missing carbs, vitamins, minerals and can lead to coronary heart disease and osteoporosis (excess protein depletes calcium)	No scientific proof; poorly controlled studies
Sugar Busters	Suggests removing all carbs from the diet	Authors are corporate CEO and three medical doctors with no nutrition backgrounds.	800–1200 Calories 0% carbs	Missing carbs, vitamins, minerals, and may cause kidney and liver damage and osteoporosis	Opinion-based; no facts
Protein Power	Claims body has no need for carbs	Michael and Mary Eades are medical doctors with no formal nutrition backgrounds.	No caloric guidelines provided but warn against letting Calories fall below 850–1000 Calories per day.	High-fat diet increases risk for coronary heart disease, high cholesterol, osteoporosis, and other health problems	No scientific research
Atkin's Diet and South Beach	Claims all carbs should be as low as possible	Dr. Robert Atkins was an MD who has touted his books since the early 60s in which some people died on this diet. He died and his company went bankrupt.	60 gram ceiling of carbs (compare this to minimal 300-gram nutritionist recommendation)	Missing carbs, vitamins, minerals and may cause kidney and liver damage, osteoporosis, and coronary artery disease from excess protein and fat	Poor company-based research
PR Nutrition	Similar claims as the Zone Diet, but catered to athletes	Dr. Sears originally started former company, but now the company denies his connection.	40% carb 30% protein 30% fat Unrestricted calories	Missing carbs, vitamins, and minerals and may cause kidney and liver damage, osteoporosis, and heart disease, especially since athletes eat more Calories. Also increases chance of "bonking" for endurance athletes.	Not research—only testimonials and athletes paid to represent their product

inform people that the testing of these foods are inconclusive and many of these foods can be eaten with other complex carb/protein/fat foods and NOT cause a reaction. Athletes and non-athletes alike will feel more satisfied with some fat in their meals and some protein (20–30 grams per meal if you eat only 3 meals a day)—see Chapter 6 regarding protein needs. If you do the calculations of an average athlete eating 3000 calories and 30% of calories coming from protein then this calculates to 225 grams of protein—higher than any amount necessary by humans in a day. The carb amount from this diet would be 300 grams—too low for an endurance athlete.

What Does Your Body Fat Percentage Mean?

The following chart gives *general* categories defining body fat percentages. This chart demonstrates that male and female bodies need differing compositions and should be used only as a tool to educate approximate guidelines and goals.

What Does Your Body Fat Percentage Mean?

Male		***Female***	
Under 3%	Not desirable; need some fat	Under 11%	Not healthy; amenorrhea
4%–10%	Elite male athletes	12%–20%	Elite female athletes
11%–15%	Fit and desirable	21%–25%	Fit and desirable
16%–20%	Typical	26%–30%	Typical
Over 24%	Considered obese	Over 33%	Considered obese

The Three Components of a Fat Loss Program

Behavior Modification for Fat Loss

For some people, knowing what to eat is not as much a problem as actually implementing the food program. Mood swings, binges, social events, and a depressed self-concept often invite unwanted eating and unwanted pounds. It is important to set realistic goals, establish mental images for yourself, practice positive affirmations and know your fender foods (those "feel-good" foods that may encourage bingeing). Find a support group of people with similar goals that can provide feedback for each other and possibly even workout together. Know what can sabotage your goals and think of strategies to avoid them (such as keeping fender foods out of the house).

Dietary Modification for Fat Loss

The old theory of weight loss still holds true for the most part: energy in = energy out. "Energy in" is the calories from food and liquid that you consume. "Energy out" is the calories expended through your basal metabolism, digestion of food, and activity. Your basal metabolism accounts for the greatest energy expended each day unless you are exercising for several hours in which your activity calories would then be greater than the metabolism calories. For example, a person who weighs 130 pounds may have a basal metabolism of about 1300 Calories (10 Calories per pound of body weight). If her daily activity Calories are 600 and the "food tax" is 190 (.10 of total calories), then the total expenditure of the day would be 2090 Calories (see Personal Assessment Estimating Energy Expenditure, Chapter 19 and Energy Metabolism, Chapter 15). Additional factors to this formula are that exercise can increase your total metabolism, fat and simple sugars tend to store as fat more easily, and the better shape you are in, the better able your body will access stored body fat for energy.

The best food strategies for weight control and fat loss are the same guidelines as those who are interested in good health and reducing their chances of disease:

> **Eat a high fiber, nutrient dense, unrefined complex carbohydrate diet with 20% of your calories coming from fats (mostly unsaturated) and moderate protein foods such as beans, plant proteins, and small amounts of low-fat animal proteins if desired. This food plan should be plentiful in fruits, veggies, and whole grains.**

Exercise Guidelines for Fat Loss

Physical activity is the magic bullet for fat loss. Exercise is the most important component of your goal to increase lean body mass and decrease body fat. Active activity will increase your exercise metabolic rate and your resting metabolic rate as well as condition the muscles and tissues. In addition, exercise will induce many positive changes in the body such as giving the body a full internal tune-up, decreasing blood fats, acting as a laxative, stimulating endorphins, increasing heart volume and work capacity, speeding healing, and decreasing depression.

The amount of exercise depends on your goals—whether they be sports-related or health-related. If you are beginning an exercise program, then think of the stair-step approach of progression. Start easy in intensity and short in duration, and then build slowly on a weekly basis. Once you have developed a foundation, then you may add more difficult workouts to your program. There has been debate over whether it is better to exercise long and slow to burn a higher percentage of body fat or to exercise short and intense to burn more calories in a shorter period of time. Exercise that is more intense will stimulate your metabolism more and will condition your heart and muscle fibers better for increasing your fitness or performance level. Including both types of exercise in your program will give you all of the above benefits as well as providing variety.

When designing your program, utilize the FITT formula:

F	**Frequency**	The number of times per week that you want to work out.	3–5 times per week of activity
I	**Intensity**	The degree of effort that you put out. Generally 60%–80% of your maximum heart rate would be appropriate.	50%–70% less intense 70%–90% more intense
T	**Time**	The length of time that you exercise.	20 minutes minimal, 40–60 minutes ideal Longer for athletes
T	**Type of activity**	Activities that you enjoy and that will contribute to your program.	Aerobic and weight training excellent for reducing body fat percentage

More details will be given for the exercise prescription in Chapter 11, Introduction for Nutrition for Sport.

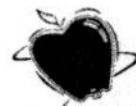

Ten Ways to Lose Body Fat and Gain Muscle

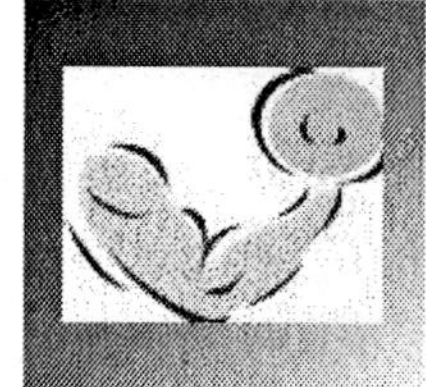

1. Exercise aerobically at least 3–4 days per week.
2. Exercise at least 30–60 minutes each time.
3. Do a variety of exercises that you enjoy.
4. Alternate slow steady with more intense workouts.
5. Include weight training in your program.
6. Eat a diet of mainly wholesome foods such as whole grains, vegetables, beans, and fruits.
7. Eat sparingly the following: meats, high-fat dairy, concentrated fats, and "junk food."
8. Limit consumption of excess sodium, cholesterol, saturated fat, total fat, and refined simple carbohydrates.
9. Measure success by how you feel or body fat testing; scales are worthless for weight loss.
10. Enjoy life, reduce stress and be nice to yourself and others!

chapter 10

Disordered Eating

What Is an Eating Disorder?

Anyone can have disordered eating when eating and food assumes an unnatural importance in his or her life, although some doctors and psychologists believe that certain conditions must be met to be medically diagnosed with an eating disorder. A person with an eating disorder (sometimes called an ED) is someone that is obsessed with food to the point of restricting food or binge eating on food. Whatever one chooses to do with food, it becomes a disorder when the behavior affects relationships, jobs, and basically one's life in a negative way. It can be an addiction in that one is not happy without this relationship with food and not happy with it. One can also develop an extremely high tolerance to foods (especially sweet foods) and consume large quantities. Eating disorders are generally divided into three categories with some overlapping characteristics.

Anorexia

Anorexia is an eating disorder that involves eating very small amounts of food and odd food rituals like counting bites of food allowed. An anorexic often wants control of her/his life and seeks to find control through food. He/she is typically from middle- to upper-income families where pressures are great to succeed.

Characteristics

1. Behavioral Signs	Signs of restricted eating (usually low intake of food) such as severe diets or fasting Odd food rituals such as counting bites of food, cutting food into tiny pieces, or preparing food for others while refusing to eat Intense fear of becoming fat, regardless of low weight Fear of food and situations where food may be present Rigid exercise regimens Dressing in layers to hide weight loss Use of laxatives, enemas, or diuretics to get rid of food; purging
2. Physiological Signs	Weight loss (often in a short period of time) (In women) cessation of menstruation without physiological cause Paleness Complaints of feeling cold Dizziness and fainting spells
3. Attitude Shifts	Mood swings Perfectionist attitude Insecurity about capabilities regardless of actual performance Feelings of self-worth being determined by what is or is not eaten Withdrawal from people

Bulimia

Bulimia ("buli" coming from the Greek meaning animalistic hunger) is an eating disorder that involves binge eating on foods and then trying to purge them in some way like exercising or vomiting or taking laxatives to rid oneself of the Calories.

Characteristics

1. Behavioral Signs	Binge eating Secretive eating, evidenced by missing food Preoccupation with and constant talk about food and/or weight The avoidance of restaurant trips, planned meals, or social events if food is present Self-disparagement when too much has been eaten Bathroom visits after meals Vomiting, laxative abuse, or fasting The use of diet pills Rigid and harsh exercise regimes Fear of being fat, regardless of weight
2. Physiological Signs	Swollen glands, puffiness in the cheeks, or broken blood vessels under the eyes Complaints of sore throats Complaints of fatigue and muscle ache Unexplained tooth decay Frequent weight fluctuations, often within a 10- to 15-pound range
3. Attitude Shifts	Mood shifts that include depression, sadness, guilt, and self-hate Severe self-criticism The need for others' approval to feel good Self-worth perceived as determined by weight

Compulsive Overeating

Compulsive overeating is the binge eating without the purging. Compulsive overeaters tend to be overweight.

Characteristics

1. Behavioral Signs	Binge eating Restriction of activities because of embarrassment about weight Going from one diet to the next Eating little in public while maintaining high weight
2. Physiological Signs	Weight-related hypertension or fatigue Weight gain
3. Attitude Shifts	Feeling about self based on weight and control of eating Fantasizing about being a better person when thin Feeling tormented by eating habits Social and professional failures attributed to weight Weight as the focus of life

What Causes an Eating Disorder?

Many people think that society causes eating disorders by its expectations of what the body should look like—especially the female body. There are many other contributing factors, however, such as early family life that included rewarding with food, force feeding, parental fears about fatness, and inaccurate parental food knowledge. Other reasons may be that the ED has learned to use food as love, relaxation, intimacy, habit, and coping with stress and that the ED has a low self-esteem. For athletes that are already susceptible, coaches can actually unintentionally bring out an eating disorder in an athlete by telling the athlete to lose weight or fat to perform better. Even subtle comments made by coaches play a major role in an athlete's decision to use desperate measures to lose weight.

The **female athlete triad** (or triple threat to female athletes) is said to be a phenomenon that is common among young female athletes, especially at the collegiate level and in those female athletes participating in appearance-based and endurance sports. The three components that affect one another are **eating disorders,** cessation of menstruation **(amenorrhea),** and **bone fractures** (ultimately osteoporosis). When a female athlete has not had menstruation for over 3 months, bone loss may be occurring no matter how much calcium is consumed. Some young female athletes with eating disorders have the curvature of the spine similar to a 70-year-old woman, and it is irreversible. Therefore, athletes who have stopped menstruating and are limiting Calories are more susceptible to bone loss, bone fractures, and long-term tissue damage and osteoporosis.

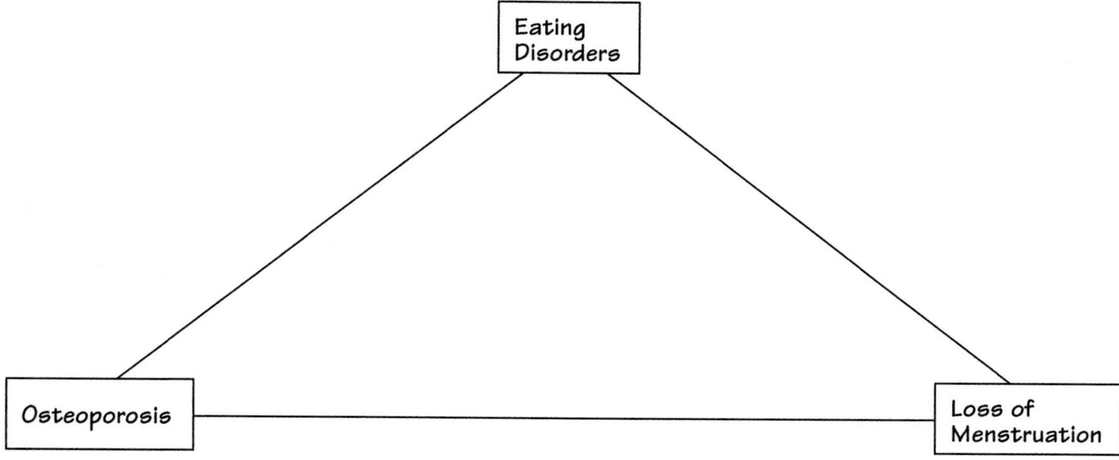

Recovery from an Eating Disorder

Just like an alcoholic, an ED is always going to be susceptible to an eating disorder, so he or she is said to always be recovering. There are many components of continuing a successful recovery. The NCAA has produced three videotapes to help coaches form a team to help the eating disordered athlete. This team may consist of the coach, a team doctor, the athletic trainer, a psychologist, a nutritionist, and the athlete. (Whoever approaches the athlete or friend needs to do so in a loving caring manner that does not include pleading or whining.) Be prepared for the ED to deny your concerns about a disorder, and have specific occurrences and behaviors that match the characteristics of the particular eating disorder.

Support groups such as Overeaters Anonymous help EDs by allowing them to hear stories of other people that have the same disorder. The goal in recovery is to help the ED find the tools to use in place of using food to deal with problems and to remain abstinent from the problem behavior. Abstinence is different for each person because an anorexic may be abstaining from starving by eating three regular meals a day, but a bulimic may be abstaining from binge eating by not going over a certain amount of food consumed. Each ED can be helped with a personal plan.

Sometimes it is necessary to supplement an anorexic's diet with a food replacement shake to add Calories until the dietary caloric intake has increased to at least 1500 calories. A nutritionist may also be able to help the ED to consume a diet that will sustain him or her and decrease the likelihood of repeated binge eating. Knowing and staying away from "fender foods"—foods that will cause a binge—is also important in early recovery. Another important tool for recovery is planning meals for the day and packing a lunch and snack to take with you. Leaving food decisions to occur when you are foodless, hungry, and away from home is usually a bad idea for any healthful food program and especially for EDs.

ED Self-Questionnaire

If you answer more than one "yes," you may have disordered eating.

	Yes	No
Do you feel guilty about eating?	______	______
Are you prone to consume large quantities of junk food?	______	______
Do you hide food or hide from others while eating?	______	______
Do you eat to the point of nausea and vomiting?	______	______
Are you sometimes repulsed by food?	______	______
Do you relish preparing foods even if you don't eat?	______	______
Have you forced vomiting?	______	______
Do you take many laxatives to control weight?	______	______
Do you weigh in on a scale more than once a week?	______	______
Have you found yourself unable to stop eating?	______	______
Have you taken on fasting to control weight?	______	______
Do you know your eating pattern is abnormal and embarrassing?	______	______
Do you eat until your stomach hurts?	______	______
Does eating cause you to fall asleep?	______	______
Do certain occasions require certain foods?	______	______
In your lifetime have you lost more than 50 pounds?	______	______
Does a "good" restaurant serve large portions?	______	______
Do you eat snacks before going out to eat with others?	______	______
Do you eat standing up?	______	______
Do you inhale your food?	______	______
Do you become irritated at postponed eating?	______	______
Have you heard others call food "too rich" and felt confused?	______	______
Do you wake from sleep to eat?	______	______
Does your wardrobe vary three sizes or more?	______	______
Does eating sometimes make you hungrier than not eating?	______	______
Do you feel like an object as others describe your body?	______	______
Have you felt people should "love me, love my fat"?	______	______
Do you usually clean your plate whether hungry or not?	______	______
Is your eating rather continual?	______	______
At a party, do you spend most of your time at the snack table, or do you consciously avoid the food area?	______	______
Have you tried more than one fad diet?	______	______
Do you make fun of others before others can?	______	______
Do you feel exhilarated when you control food?	______	______
Are you afraid to be "normal"?	______	______
When you know certain foods are on the shelf, do they "call" to you?	______	______
Do you buy clothes either too big or too small?	______	______
Do your friends eat like you or are they embarrassed?	______	______
Do you postpone joys with "wait 'til I control my weight"?	______	______
Do others see your shape differently than you do?	______	______

chapter 11

Introduction to Nutrition for Sport and Exercise

This entire book is a practical approach of nutrition for lifelong optimal health and fitness. This chapter expands on nutrition for fitness and health and also introduces the topic of sports nutrition in which athletes are striving to find the nutritional edge in competition and sport. *Establish fitness lifestyles early.*

Starting to Exercise

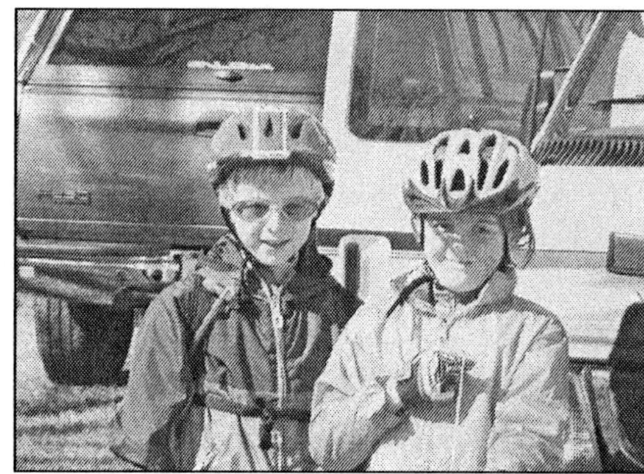

There are many benefits of engaging in physical activity such as improving cardiovascular health, maintaining lean muscle tissue, reducing health risks associated with obesity, enhancing insulin action, strengthening bones, reducing susceptibility to infections, reducing cancer risk, improving peristaltic functions, getting fewer injuries, and improving psychological health. In addition, nutrition influences physical performance and nutrient use. However, only 15% of adults are regularly physically active!

When you want to begin an exercise program, do the following.

- Start out slowly
- Vary your workout; make it fun
- Include others to help you keep accountable
- Set attainable goals
- Set aside specific time
- Focus on the long term and not on occasional setbacks

As you begin to design your workout or training program you will want to consider various training principles and developing all aspects of health-related physical fitness:

- Flexibility (stretching)
- Strength (resistance training)
- Muscular endurance (repetition work with the muscles)
- Cardiovascular endurance (aerobic exercise working the heart)
- Body composition (ratio of body fat to lean body mass)

As you are creating your own fitness plan, the principles of conditioning will help you to train smartly to prevent injury and overuse and to improve your overall fitness more efficiently:

- **Overload Principle**—The main concept of physical training where you place a greater stress on the body than was previously endured.
- **Progressive Resistance Exercise** (PRE)—Resistance is increased as you adapt to each level; primarily in weight training, but can be applied to athletic training workouts.
- **Specificity Principle**—Physical training should be designed to mimic the same specific athletic event or activity that you are training for.

The Physical Activity Pyramid Depicts General Health-Related Fitness Guidelines

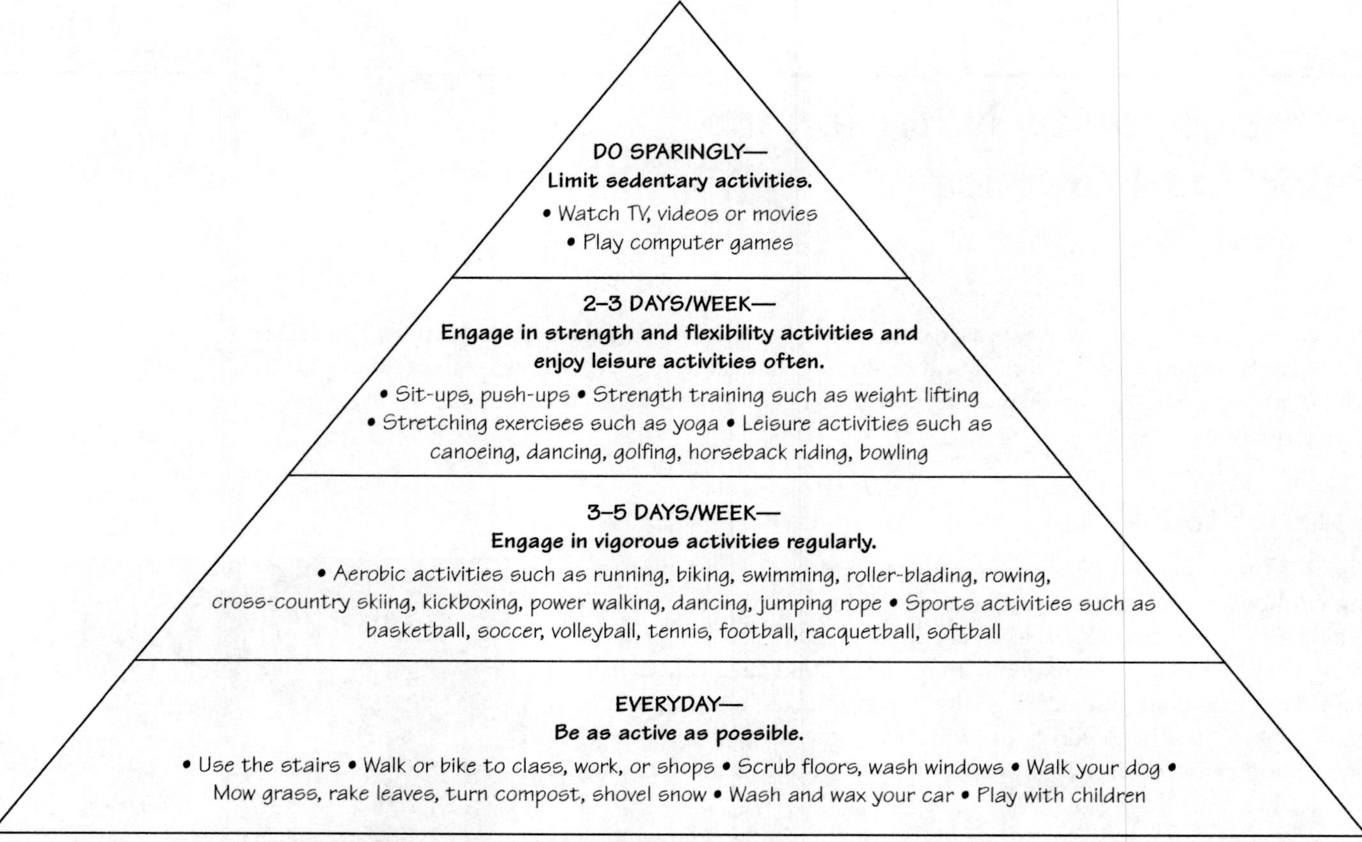

Adapted from Corbin, C.B. and Lindsey, R. 2004. *Fitness for Life, Fifth Edition.* Champaign, IL: Human Kinetics Publishers. May not be reproduced without permission of Human Kinetics.

- **Recuperation Principle**—Adequate rest periods are taken for recuperation such as the hard/easy regimen of keeping recovery days in-between hard days for specific muscle groups (i.e., spinning in an easy gear on the bike for recovery the day following hill repeat intervals).

The **FITT** formula was introduced in chapter 9:

F	Frequency	The number of times per week that you want to work out.	3–5 times per week of activity
I	Intensity	The degree of effort that you put out. Generally 60%–80% of your maximum heart rate would be appropriate.	50%–70% less intense 70%–90% more intense
T	Time	The length of time that you exercise.	20 minutes minimal 40–60 minutes ideal Longer for athletes
T	Type of Activity	Activities that you enjoy and that will contribute to your program.	Aerobic and weight training excellent for reducing body fat %

In chapter 19 you will be able to design your own fitness program for the elements of health-related fitness using the principles of conditioning and the FITT formula.

Helpful Training Charts

The following charts will assist you in establishing your goals. See chapter 9 for more information about the FITT formula.

	Week	Heart rate Intensity	Duration (min)	Freq (∞/wk)
Initial Phase	1	50%	10	3
	2	60%	10	3
	3	70%	15	3
	4	70%–75%	15	4
	5	75%–80%	20	4
Improvement Phase	6–9	75%–80%	20	4
	10–16	80%	25–30	4
	17–23	80%	30	4–5
	24–27	80%	30	4–6
Maintenance Phase	28+	80%	40–60	4–6

Source: Zaret, B. L., M. Moser and L. S. Cohen, Eds. *Yale University Heart Book.* New York: Hearst Books, 1992.

Target Heart Rate Zones (50%–80% Threshold) According to Age

RHR	Age							
	30–34	35–39	40–44	45–49	50–54	55–59	60–64	65–69
45–59	118–167	115–163	113–158	110–154	108–150	105–146	103–141	100–137
50–54	120–168	117–164	115–159	112–155	110–151	107–147	105–142	102–138
55–59	123–168	120–164	118–159	115–155	113–151	110–147	108–142	105–138
60–64	125–169	122–165	120–160	117–156	115–152	112–148	110–143	107–139
65–69	128–170	125–166	123–161	122–157	118–153	115–149	113–144	110–140
70–74	130–171	127–167	125–162	124–158	120–154	117–150	115–145	112–141
75–79	133–172	130–168	128–163	125–159	123–155	120–151	118–146	115–142
80–84	135–173	132–169	130–164	127–160	125–156	122–152	120–146	117–143

Note: RHR is resting heart rate.

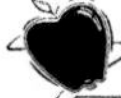

Recommendations for Improving Muscular Strength and Endurance

	# Sets	# Reps	Sessions/ Wk	# of Exercises	Overall Purpose
ACSM	1	8–12	2	8–10	Basic development and maintenance of fat-free mass
Cooper Institute					
Minimum	1	8–12	2	10	Strength maintenance
Recommended	2	8–12	2	10	Strength improvement
Optimal	3	8–12	2	10	Noticeable gains in strength

Basic Energy Metabolism

The chemical energy current used by cells for muscle contractions is ATP (adenosine triphosphate). Only a small amount of ATP is stored in resting cells (for 2–4 sec. of work), therefore, other sources of energy are needed. Phosphocreatine, carbohydrates, fats, protein, and some by-products of metabolism will provide energy to be metabolized within three basic energy systems of the body. The following chart lists the three energy systems and their characteristics.

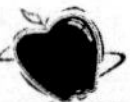

Phosphocreatine (PCr)	***Anaerobic Glycolysis***	***Aerobic Glycolysis***
A high-energy compound formed and stored in the muscle	Limited oxygen during intense physical activity (sprinting)	Plenty of oxygen available for low to moderate intensity
Not enough stored in the muscle to sustain ATP for more than a few minutes (generally useful for the first 10–15 seconds)	3 carbon pyruvate is converted to lactate; produces 2 ATP per glucose and lactate buildup changing acidity and inhibiting glycolysis enzymes	Produces 36–38 ATP per glucose (95% of energy potential) and provides energy for 2 minutes to 3 hours of work
Activated instantly and replenishes ATP	Replenishes ATP quickly and provides energy for 30 seconds to 2 minutes of work	Replenishes ATP slowly

Some tips on your Preendurance Event Meal

- Consumed 2–4 hours prior to event
- Consist primarily of CHO (top off glycogen)
- Low fat
- Little fiber if not used to (prevent bloating, gas)
- Moderate or low protein
- Avoid fatty, fried foods
- Blended or liquid meal can be consumed 1–2 hrs prior

The Active Body's Use of Fuels—Carbs

Carbohydrate is the crucial nutrient for active people, provided by the liver, muscle tissue, and blood in the form of glucose and glycogen. *Aerobic* activity will conserve glycogen stores to some extent, and *Anaerobic* activity will rapidly use glycogen stores. The longer the activity, the more glycogen depleted so eventually carbohydrate must be replenished along with fluids.

The body is able to temporarily store glucose in the liver and muscle. Glycogen is the storage form of carbohydrates in the liver and muscle. Muscle glycogen is used only by that muscle; liver glycogen is released into the bloodstream. Some important points about carbohydrates are the following:

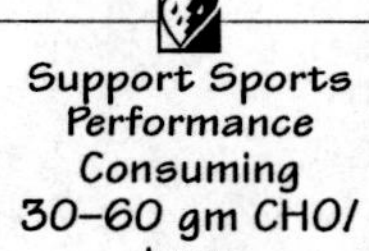

Support Sports Performance Consuming 30–60 gm CHO/ hour

- Fresh or dried fruit
- Energy bars such as Clif or Powerbar
- Gels such as GU or Powergel
- Sports drinks such as Endura or Cytomax

- At low to moderate intensity; they will sustain work for up to about 2 hours.
- Once glycogen is depleted, you can only work at ~50% of maximal capacity ("bonking").
- Workouts will train specific muscles to maximize glycogen stores.
- Blood glucose is an important source of fuel.
- An intake of 30–60 gm CHO/hour is helpful during strenuous endurance activity.
- Carbohydrate consumption during exercise delays fatigue.
- Carbohydrate is the main fuel for all types of activity.
- Consume at least 60% of your total Calories from carbohydrates.
- Adhere to the food guide pyramids or Healthful House of Food and Fitness.
- For aerobic and endurance training and preparation, consume 6–10 gm of carbohydrate (CHO)/ kg body weight.
- Marathoners consume about 500–700 gm of CHO/day (see chapter 16).

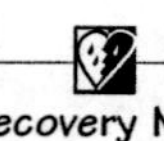

Recovery Meal

- Consumed within 2 hours (preferably 1 hour) after endurance event
- CHO rich (1.5 g/kg body weight) to replace glycogen
- Repeat CHO meal over the next 2-hour interval
- Aim for 4:1 CHO to protein ratio
- Remember to consume fluids and electrolytes, too

Follow a modern glycogen-loading regimen for events lasting longer than 60–90 minutes to maximize glycogen stores by tapering exercise while increasing CHO intake. Additional water weight will be gained since glycogen stores water. Carbo loading is explained in detail in chapter 16, "Healthful Nutrition for Training and Competition."

The Active Body's Use of Fuels—Fats and Fatty Acids

The *longer* the exercise, the *more* fat percent of Calories will be burned (20 min. is often the minimum time to begin fat cell shrinkage). The *slower* the activity, the *greater percent* of fat burned (50% fat/50% glycogen for ultramarathon). More *trained* muscles will burn a *higher fat percent* over glycogen and

A Minor Source of Fuel

- Provides only 2%–5% of energy needs during rest and low/moderate exercise
- Provides 10%–15% of energy needs during endurance exercise
- Most energy from branched-chain amino acids
- A carbohydrate-rich diet spares protein from being used as fuel

have more mitochondria to utilize fat as fuel. Fat recommendations for active people and athletes are similar to sedentary people, with the exception for sometimes a higher intake of "good" fats for caloric density when needed.

Fat for Athletes

- 20%–30% of total kcal (35% max)
- Rich in MUFA
- Limit saturated fats
- Limit hydrogenated fats

The Active Body's Use of Fuels—Proteins

Although protein has many important functions listed in chapter 6, protein does not provide a large percentage of the fuel needed for activity. Athletes need a little more protein per kilogram of body weight, which can be obtained through eating whole foods.

Energy (Caloric) Needs of Active People and Athletes

Energy needs can be estimated by scientific measurements of indirect and direct calorimetry, but the most practical means is to monitor body composition in relation to weight and set formulas (see personal assessment worksheet). A desirable body fat for male athletes is 5%–18% whereas a desirable body fat for female athletes is 17%–28%. In general, if your weight falls, increase intake of kcal. If body fat increases, cut back in fat (and kcal) and maintain activity. To gain muscle you need rest, resistance exercise, and increased kilocalories (see chapter 18 for more details on muscle gain). Some athletes such as wrestlers are encouraged to "make weight" the wrong way while losing weight to qualify for a lower weight class. Many will lose pounds by diuretics leading to dehydration, then dehydration adversely affects their performance. These practices can increase the risk for kidney malfunction, heart problems, and death. The National Collegiate Athletic Association is encouraging wrestlers to "make weight" the right way by requiring a minimum safe weight set by a physician or trainer and a gradual reduction in food intake long before competition.

Protein for Athletes

- Recommend 1.2 gm protein/kg body weight (up from typical .8)
- Sometimes up to 1.4 grams for individuals participating in endurance exercise
- Needs are easily met by a normal diet
- Protein supplements are not necessary
- Excessive protein has not been shown to be beneficial

Vitamins and Minerals for Activity

Most of the vitamin and mineral DRIs that have been established to cover the needs of most active people. Athletes sometimes need a little extra of specific vitamins and minerals, and these needs may easily be satisfied by consuming whole foods such as emphasized in the Healthful House of Food and Fitness (vegetables, fruits, whole grains, legumes, nuts, and seeds). Athletes may need a slightly higher intake of vitamin E and vitamin C (for their antioxidant properties in repairing tissue damage). They may also need extra thiamin, riboflavin, vitamin B_6, potassium, magnesium, iron, zinc, copper, and chromium because of their role in metabolism. Iron intake and deficiency symptoms can be monitored because an iron deficiency will affect performance. *Sports anemia*, however, may occur due to the increase in plasma volume but this is not true anemia. Women are at risk for iron deficiency because of menstruation, so be sure to focus on iron-rich foods (see plant sources in chapter 7). Calcium is another specific mineral of concern when there is a restriction of Calories (especially by women). Calcium deficiency or calcium excretion will compromise bone health. In addition, amenorrhea (loss of menstruation) will affect bone density and possibly lead to osteoporosis (see chapter 10, Disordered Eating). Extra calcium does not compensate for amenorrhea.

Fluid Needs

The average person needs 1 ml/kcal fluid per day which is equivalent to ~8 C per day for the average adult consuming 2000 Calories per day. Athletes need this and more since fluids are needed to maintain body's cooling system during exercise. Athletes who lose more than 3% of body weight during exercise will likely experience hindered performance.

Three major heat illnesses can occur when your body fluid losses are not replenished.

Hydration Tips for the Athlete

- Thirst is not a reliable indicator of fluid needs.
- Drink 2–3 C of fluids per pound of weight loss during activity.
- Drink fluid freely 24 hours before the event.
- Drink 1.5–2.5 C two–three hours before the event.
- Drink 1/2–1 1/2 C every 15 minutes for events longer than 30 min.

Characteristics of **heat exhaustion** include

- A depletion of blood volume from fluid loss by the body
- Body heat is lost primarily through evaporation of sweat
- Fluid loss through sweat is about 3–8 C per hour
- Humidity interferes with sweat production
- Decreases endurance, strength, performance
- Profuse sweating, headache, dizziness, nausea, weakness, visual disturbances

Characteristics of **heat cramps** include

- Occurs in the skeletal muscle
- A complication of heat exhaustion
- Painful muscle contractions for 1–3 minutes at a time
- Ensure athletes have adequate salt and fluid intake
- Exercise moderately at first in the heat to prevent

Characteristics of **heat stroke** include

- Internal body temperature reaches 105°F
- Symptoms: nausea, confusion, irritability, poor coordination, seizures, and coma
- Athletes should replace fluids and monitor weight change (fluid loss)
- Avoid exercising under hot, humid conditions

Fluid replacement (also called "Sports" or "Glucose Polymer") **drinks** may be used for endurance exercise > 60 minutes. The sweat, CHO, and electrolytes lost in events < 60 minutes are easily replaced by diet, but in events > 60 minutes a sports drink can help maintain the blood glucose level and blood volume. The carbohydrate concentration of a sports drink that is best absorbed is 6%, which is 15 grams of carbohydrate per cup of the mixed fluid (see chapter 17 for more fluid details for athletes).

Ergogenic Aids

Athletes have tried many substances of all types to try to enhance sports performance. See chapter 16 for a detailed chart.

chapter 12

Safety Issues and World Concerns in Nutrition

Food Safety Issues

Many people are concerned with the safety of their foods and worried that they can get sick or damaged. Such concerns include pesticides, hormones, bacteria, viruses, chemical additives, and toxic metals. Food-borne illness is a major cause of diarrhea. There is usually no real long-term health threat to the average person, but it may be serious for very young, very old, and people with long-term illness. Food-borne illness usually results from unsafe food handling in the **home.** Microbes are able to produce specific toxins that can invade the intestinal wall, produce an infection, and be intoxicating. Food tends to make us sick more these days because of the preference for "rare" meats, use of immunity suppressant medications, increase in the number of elderly, increase in the shelf life of products, which allows for bacterial growth, and an increase in the consumption of imported ready-to-eat foods. People are constantly at risk for **food-borne** illness.

Irradiation Logo on Food

Ways Industry Trys to Reduce Food-Borne Illness

The food industry tries to reduce food poisoning by the use of food preservation such as using salt, sugar, smoke, fermentation, and drying techniques that will prevent the growth of bacteria and limit the water available for bacteria. Pasteurization, sterilization, refrigeration, freezing, irradiation, canning, chemical preservation, and aseptic processing are all techniques the industry utilizes to reduce bacterial growth. A controversial food preservation technique is food **irradiation** that does not make food radioactive, but breaks down chemical bonds, cell walls, and DNA that will control and limit the growth of bacteria. The FDA considers irradiation to be safe and has approved it to be used on raw meats. However, irradiation causes the loss of vitamins and emits radiolytic by-products that may affect our health negatively.

Reducing Your Own Chances of Sickness as a Consumer

You can prevent food-borne illness at the store by getting frozen, perishable foods last, placing meats in separate plastic bags, avoiding dented cans, buying only pasteurized milk/cheese, buying only what you need, and steering clear of slimy, brownish, dry produce. You can prevent food-borne illnesses during preparation by washing hands thoroughly; keeping counters, cutting boards, and equipment clean and sanitized; preparing raw meat on a separate cutting board, thawing foods in refrigerator or cold running water or microwave; avoiding coughing and sneezing over food; and cleaning and washing fruits and vegetables thoroughly. Ground meats should be consumed within 1–2 days from the refrigerator and frozen meat used within 3–4 months. The Food Safety Motto is **"When in doubt, throw it out!"** When cooking, be sure to thoroughly cook meat, fish, poultry, and eggs. Cook stuffing separately, consume food right away, store "leftovers" within 2 hours, serve cooked meat on clean plates, and avoid partially cooking food for picnics. Take special care with leftovers to keep hot foods hot and cold foods cold (< 40° F or > 140° F), reheat leftovers to 165° F, and store peeled, cut-up produce in the refrigerator. There are also dangers of cross contamination from one contaminated source to clean source and from unclean hands to food. You should practice sanitary food handling at home and expect the same practice when eating out.

The following shows the temperature danger zone.

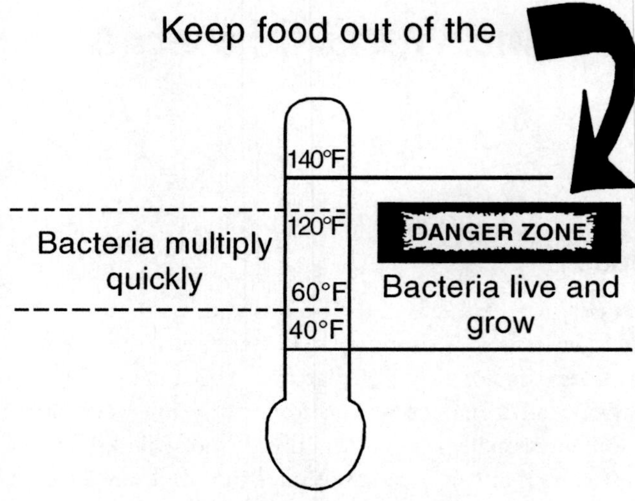

Additives

Additives are added to food to limit spoilage and prevent undesirable changes. However, the safety is sometimes questionable. **Intentional** food additives are added directly to food, **incidental** food additives find their way into food on their own (hair and bugs), and sometimes additives are indirectly added as a contaminant (i.e., pesticide residue). The FDA regulates additives and has established the GRAS (Generally Recognized as Safe) List for additives generally regarded as safe. Therefore, manufacturers do not have to prove their safety, but if it is shown to cause cancer even at a high dose, it is taken off the market (Delaney Clause). Some common food additives are the following:

- Acid or alkaline agents
- Alternative sweeteners
- Anticaking agents
- Antimicrobial agents
- Antioxidants
- Colors
- Emulsifiers
- Flavor enhancers
- Nutrient supplements
- Curing and pickling agents

There are also natural toxins and chemicals in foods such as *solanine* from potato shoots, *mushroom toxins*, *advidin* in raw egg whites, *thiaminase* in raw clams and mussels, *protease inhibitor* in raw soybeans, and various ones found in *herbal teas.*

Toxic Metals in Foods

Toxic metals contaminate food and our environment and can be life threatening. **Lead** is a heavy toxic metal that can cause anemia and kidney disease and damage the nervous system. Lead comes from solder joints, lead paint, playgrounds, and metal containers. A high-fat, low-calcium, low-iron diet absorbs more lead, therefore, a low-fat, adequate calcium and iron diet is recommended. **Mercury** accumulates in the fish that is mainly consumed by large predator fish such as shark and swordfish. These fish are tested more frequently for mercury levels. Women of childbearing years should limit fish intake because of their common association with birth defects. **Urethane** is from fermentation of alcohol that increases upon the heating of the alcohol. It causes cancer in animal studies.

Genetically Engineered Foods

Genetic engineering is the process of artificially tampering with DNA blueprints where scientists insert the gene of one organism into another in an effort to replicate characteristics in the receiving organism. So, for example, genetic engineers have added genes from the flounder to tomatoes in an attempt to give tomatoes a longer shelf life. Genetic engineers also plan to use the technology to improve nutrition and even come up with medical benefits. But some biotechnology companies are also using genetic engineering to produce crops that can withstand increased amounts of pesticides, often pesticides sold by those very same companies. Genetic engineering is such a new technology that no one's sure what the health consequences might be, and it may take years to find out. Just like in one of the other great food revolutions of the twentieth century, scientists didn't realize the health consequences of heavy agricultural pesticide usage until years after pesticides were introduced. In 1999, Cornell scientists discovered that genetically engineered corn might be deadly to the monarch butterfly. That's just the tip of the iceberg when it comes to environmental concerns. When biotech corporations boast that genetic engineering can do wonders for the environment, consider the source. After all, some of these companies are the same ones that have invented such deadly pesticides such as DDT and Agent Orange. These pesticides, it was promised, would help the environment, yet they turned into environmental disasters. One of the best (and only) ways to avoid genetically engineered foods in the United States is to eat organically grown food. Organic foods are regarded by many people as more nutritious and delicious than their nonorganic counterparts. Unfortunately, genetically engineered foods are creating a number of problems for organic growers.

Organic Standards and Labeling

Organic farming was one of the fastest growing segments of U.S. agriculture during the 1990s and continues to grow.

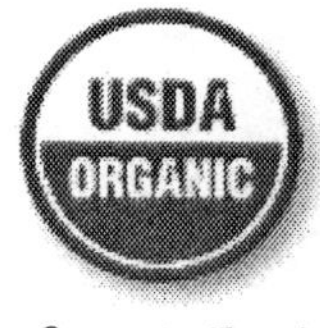

Organic Food Logo

The National Organic Standards Board Definition of "Organic"

The following definition of "organic" was passed by the NOSB at its April 1995 meeting in Orlando, Florida.

> Organic agriculture is an ecological production management system that promotes and enhances biodiversity, biological cycles and soil biological activity. It is based on minimal use of off-farm inputs and on management practices that restore, maintain and enhance ecological harmony.
>
> "Organic" is a labeling term that denotes products produced under the authority of the Organic Foods Production Act. The principal guidelines for organic production are to use materials and practices that enhance the ecological balance of natural systems and that integrate the parts of the farming system into an ecological whole.
>
> Organic agriculture practices cannot ensure that products are completely free of residues; however, methods are used to minimize pollution from air, soil and water.
>
> Organic food handlers, processors and retailers adhere to standards that maintain the integrity of organic agricultural products. The primary goal of organic agriculture is to optimize the health and productivity of interdependent communities of soil life, plants, animals and people.

Reduce Your Exposure to Toxins

Know what foods pose a risk for food poisoning (meat, poultry, dairy, eggs, and fish), practice moderation and variety, trim fat from meat and fish, wash fruits and vegetables thoroughly, buy organic, and cook meat thoroughly.

World Nutrition Concerns

Hunger and sustainability issues are at the forefront of current global concerns. Almost half of the world's population earns less than $200 a year, and 80%–90% of that income is spent on food. One in eight people in the United States is going to bed hungry. Today 790 million people are malnourished in the world.

Nutrients that are often missing worldwide are iron, iodine, and vitamin A. Undernutrition can begin during pregnancy when a pregnant woman's needs are higher. Undernutrition affects fetal development and can result in the death of the woman and/or the child. Women in Africa give birth to an average of 6 live babies. Undernutrition during the fetal period and infancy can cause poor growth and development, preterm delivery, reduced lung development, and long-term health problems. Undernutrition during childhood can lead to permanent brain impairment, stunted growth, impaired motor skills, and low resistance to infection. This is a period of rapid growth rate, especially for the brain and CNS (central nervous system). Undernutrition during the older years can cause low resistance to infection and may be the result of a fixed income and a forced choice between medication and food. Nutrient-dense foods are required.

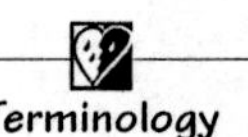

Terminology

- *Hunger:* physiological state when not enough food is eaten to meet energy needs
- *Malnutrition:* condition of impaired development or function caused by deficiency
- *Undernutrition:* limited food supply to meet the needs of a population
- *Overnutrition:* excess amount of food leading to overconsumption and poor food choices
- *Famine:* extreme shortage of food leading to massive starvation in a population

The Historical Perspective of Hunger

The Depression was an era of profound hunger. Pellagra and rickets spread from undernutrition of vitamins. The government created federally funded soup kitchens; the school lunch program (1946), the food stamp program, and the school breakfast program for low-income persons (1965); and developed congregate meals and meals-on-wheels. Since this time, there has been expansion of the food stamp program, expansion of the school lunch and breakfast programs, and the creation of Women, Infants, and Children (WIC) in 1972. Currently federal funds fall short, there are not enough jobs available, and eligibility and funding for federal programs is tightened. Privately funded programs have also been developed to combat hunger.

Socioeconomic Factors Related to Undernutrition

Poverty is the result of large group unskilled workers, massive layoffs, low-paying service jobs, and an increase in the number of single-parent families. Homelessness is widespread, with 43% of homeless families with children, cost of housing increased, subsidy for housing decreased, and the widespread release of mentally ill patients from institutions. Difficulties that confront the poor are substandard education, poor skills, lack of reliable and safe child care, inability to relocate, little employment experience, and limited financial reserve to fall back on.

The Solution

All Americans are affected by the hunger problem, either directly or indirectly, and the solution requires a cultural shift emphasizing the responsibility of individuals. You can donate your time, money, and/or food; exercise your right to vote; and write and/or e-mail your congresspersons. Some obstacles that exist in developing countries are extreme imbalances in food/population ratio, war and political/civil unrest, rapid depletion of natural resources, some cultural attitudes towards certain foods, poor infrastructure, and debt.

Population Problem

With the increasing growth of the population, which is exceeding economic growth, there is an increase in poverty, and disparities exist between the rich and poor in regards to access and affordability of food. It is estimated that by 2030, 9 out of 10 infants will be born in the poorest parts of the world. Economists estimate that there will be enough food produced to meet the needs of the increasing population until the year 2020, but distribution may be a problem. Because of population growth, food production will probably begin to lag behind population growth by the year of 2025. Poorer people are bearing more children because larger family size ensures longevity of the family. The poorer countries are increasing their population the most, and often cultural and religious beliefs conflict with birth control programs. Women in the United States have an average of 2.1 live births, whereas East African countries average 8.5 live births per woman. The average worldwide is 4.0 live births per woman. In response to the population problem in China, where 22% of the world's population lives, the Chinese government allows one child per urban couple and allows for two children in rural areas only if the first child is a girl. The current birthrate is 1.8 per woman, and penalties are placed on having extra children. This tends to be a program successful for population control, but controversial for values.

Other factors contributing to worldwide hunger are war and political unrest that causes an increase in global military spending. Civil disruptions and war contribute to undernutrition, and political divisions may impede distribution of food. War destroys food production and infrastructure and contributes to a depletion of natural resources.

Undernutrition in the United States

- ~50 million Americans live at or near poverty level.
- Poverty is defined as an annual income of $16,050 for a family of four.
- ~50% of the poor are children.
- Choice between food, rent, or heat.
- More related to politics and socioeconomic than scarcity of food.

Contamination

The population and supply problems are major factors in the web of interconnected global environmental issues that exists. However, contamination of our waters, land, and food is equally a concern. Seventy-five of all diseases (one-third of all deaths) are related to the consumption of contaminated water. The WHO (World Health Organization) issued a statement that breastfeeding in third-world countries would eliminate many of these deaths. Human urine and feces are dangerous contaminants that contaminate water. Bovine feces is a worldwide contamination problem resulting in nitrites in the water supply. The livestock in the United States produce 20 times as much excrement as the entire human population of the country.

Agribusiness Issues

Countries are spending more than they make and borrowing money from foreign countries. Many are on the verge of economic collapse. This places a burden on developing countries and limits their ability to implement programs to reduce undernutrition.

How to Reduce Undernutrition in the Developing Countries

You can reduce undernutrition by giving direct food aid, although not a long-term solution, and/or by joining the Peace Corps to provide education, distribute food and medical supplies, create independent, self-sustaining economies, and create a sustainable food environment. Ending female neglect is also an important step in reducing undernutrition. Women make up 70% of people worldwide living in poverty, work longer hours than men, and grow food for family consumption. There is a grand need to provide women with education and political power. We can also end world hunger by the supplementation of indigenous foods with nutrients, providing education and training to become self-sufficient, raising the economic status, increasing the availability of food, and encouraging political cooperation.

The "Green Revolution"

Sustainable agriculture is a must for the future of the world. The exploitation of earth can only go so far. More people can be fed on a plant-based diet—read **Frances Moore Lappe's** *Diet for Small Planet* (most of the grain produced in our country goes to the cattle instead of people). According to **John Robbins** of the Earth Save Foundation, what you eat has the greatest impact of all on the environment and the future of our planet. Read *Diet for a New America, May All Be Fed*, and *The Food Revolution: How Your Diet Can Help Save Your Life and Our World* for details about how our meat, dairy products, and egg consumption uses the most resources, land, and water in the United States and is a leading polluter of the environment, as well as contributing to the leading cause of death in the United States. For a sustainable agriculture, the farmer can rotate crops, use beneficial insects, decrease pesticide use, and work toward organic farming methods. The consumer can buy organic and eat less animal foods. It is up to **you**, and **you** can make a difference!

chapter 13

Life-Cycle Nutrition—Gravida, Infant, Child, and the Aging

Gravida (a pregnant woman) nutrition is a critical component of prenatal care as well as blood analysis and optional testing, monitoring, exercise guidelines, and pregnancy and lactation education. Be sure to choose a midwife or doctor that will allow you to take control of your pregnancy—ask lots of questions and know what you want.

Pregnancy and Gestation

A full-term gestational period is **38–42 weeks** so babies are not born "early" or "late" if they are within these weeks. A preterm or premature baby is one born prior to full term (generally prior to 37 weeks). The pregnancy or gestational period is divided into **trimesters,** or three 13-week periods. The term for the little human is an **embryo** for 2 to 8 weeks and a **fetus** from 8 weeks to birth. Some common pregnancy terms are **LBW** for low birth weight (under 5.5 pounds) and **SGA** for small for gestational age (full term, but less than 5.5 pounds).

"Morning Sickness" and Cravings

As hormonal changes occur during pregnancy, most women experience some sort of nausea, often labeled "morning" sickness, although it can occur any time of the day. The theory behind the "morning" label is that in earlier days husbands were seeing their wives sick in the morning then leaving for work, thereby saying their wives had "morning" sickness. Generally the nausea (and sometimes vomiting) ends after the first trimester, but some women, although rare, experience severe vomiting the entire pregnancy (hyperemesis gravidarum). The fetus utilizes a great amount of glucose from the mother's blood so some of the nausea results from the mother's blood sugar falling too low. Some morning sickness solutions are making healthful dietary choices and avoiding foods that make you nauseated to smell. **Gingerroot** is an herb that has been used in the form of teas and ginger products to reduce nausea. Sucking on a **lemon** has also been found to be helpful for relieving nauseas, as well as supplementing with **B_6** for extreme sickness. Women who exercise regularly and moderately tend to experience less sickness. Get lots of rest, wake up slowly in the morning, keep a wholesome carbohydrate-rich snack handy for middle of the night snacking (i.e., Trader Joe's tofu cheese on whole-grain crackers), and use common sense in avoiding "fender" smells (those that will make you sick, such as coffee, gasoline, perfume, cleaning products, trash, and greasy foods).

Some women will experience **pica** during pregnancy, which is the craving for nonfood substances, such as dirt and clay, and there are even case studies of the consumption of toilet bowl freshener and tire tubes.

Weight Breakdown (25–35 pounds):

- 7–8 pounds baby
- 1–2 pounds placenta
- 2–3 pounds breast
- 4 pounds blood
- 2 pounds fluid
- 2 pounds uterus

Weight Gain During Pregnancy

In the 1950s women were discouraged from gaining more than 15 pounds during pregnancy, then in the 1970s it was considered "healthy" to gain 50 or 60 pounds. The current recommendation for gravida weight gain is 25–35 pounds (more if overly lean before conception and less if overly fat prior to pregnancy).

Exercise and Pregnancy

Women who moderately exercise tend to have babies with increased birth weights compared to sedentary gravidas. The recommendation for exercise during pregnancy is to be able to talk while exercising (not be too anaerobic), consume plenty of fluids, avoid exercising in extreme heat (102 degree internal limit), and do not do more exercise than you were doing before pregnancy. Stretching, Kegals (pelvic strengthening exercises), hiking, and swimming are all excellent gravida exercises, and be sure to stay away from contact sports!

Increased Needs/ Changes in the RDA
- Energy: + 300 Calories
- Protein: + 10–15 grams
- Zinc: + 3 mg
- **Folate: 600 mcg**
- **Iron: 27 mg**

Nutrient Needs Increase

Some nutrient needs are higher for a gravida as listed in the DRI charts. Nutrient needs are even higher for lactating women. Iron and folate needs increase the most.

Supplementation and Nutrient-Dense Food Sources

Supplementation is not necessary if nutrient-dense foods are consumed, but the extra insurance of supplementation is not a bad idea during pregnancy, as long as vitamin A levels are less than 5000 IU in the supplement to avoid a toxicity amount leading to malformations and birth defects. Vitamin A is teratogenic and must be avoided in excess amounts. Vegetarian gravidas have the same nutrient requirements and can meet their nutrient needs with nutrient-dense sources as well. The fetus will get its **nourishment** provided by the **placenta**, the organ that grows only during pregnancy in the woman's body and transfers oxygen and nutrients to the fetus with a blood barrier between the fetal and maternal side of the placenta. The fetus will take what it needs, and if the gravida is deficient then the gravida will suffer first.

Nutritious Food Sources during Pregnancy
- *Folate:* Lentils, beans, dark greens, OJ
- *Iron:* Whole grains, beans, peas, prunes, blackstrap molasses, dried fruit
- *Zinc:* Nuts, greens, whole grains
- *Calcium:* Beans, greens, almond butter, sesame seeds, fortified soy and rice milks, soy cheese, sea veggies, corn tortillas, dried figs

Special Concerns During Pregnancy

Fetal alcohol syndrome and spina bifida are preventable outcomes of pregnancies that affect the infant. Even a small amount of alcohol can cause permanent mental and physical malformations as well as a much smaller brain in the infant. These characteristics, when diagnosed, add up to **FAS**. Fetal alcohol effects is when the infant has some of the characteristics, but not all of them and is from the mom drinking during pregnancy. Spina bifida occurs when there is an inadequate amount of folate in the gravida's diet. The neural tube does not form properly, and the baby may be paralyzed for life or die. If the gravida consumes alcohol, smokes cigarettes, takes other drugs, is exposed to environmental contaminants or food additives, or receives too much vitamin A in the retinol form, then she may experience premature rupture of the membranes (PROM), an LBW baby, or a baby with malformations and birth defects. Caffeine consumption during pregnancy may decrease iron absorption, reduce blood flow through the placenta, increase risk of spontaneous abortion (heavy caffeine use), increase risk of a low-birth-weight infant, and cause missing digits. A general recommendation is to limit caffeine intake (< 2 cups coffee/day).

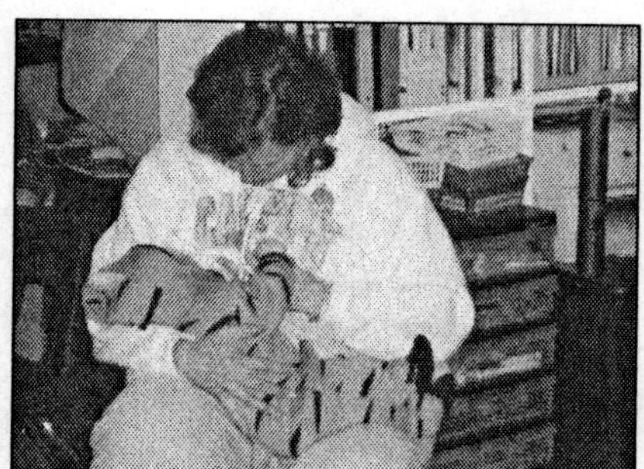

Infant and Child Nutrition

From Breastfeeding to Solids

Whether you were breastfed as a child and whether you or your partner will breastfeed, as well as how long you breastfeed and how you feel about breastfeeding in public largely depends on where you were born and the cultural and social influences surrounding you. In the late 1800s, 90% of women breastfed their babies and did not wean them until them were ready, which was after 2 years of age. Now in the year of 2000 less than half of women breastfeed, and they wean before the baby is 6 months old. The book *Breastfeeding: Biocultural Perspectives*, by Katherine Dettwyler, attempts to fill the gap between the bicultural crisis that exists with breastfeeding today. Check out 101 Reasons to Breastfeed at www.promom.org for many advantages of breastfeeding.

Working and Breastfeeding

A woman who still needs to or desires to work can often find ways to be with the baby for feedings such as taking the baby with her, having the baby close to where she works for frequent feedings, or have the baby brought to her for feedings. A mother can also pump milk every 2–3 hours during work and store in the refrigerator to be given by childcare provider by cup or bottle while she is separated from the baby. Because ~99% of women can breastfeed, most women who choose to feed artificial milk have not been educated about breastfeeding and its vital benefits or they are just doing what their mothers did. Make sure to get training if you bottle-feed artificial milk such as wearing a mask for sickness, and keeping lot numbers for frequent recalls. Avoid giving the baby a bottle to go to sleep, as this will cause baby bottle tooth decay (does not happen from breastfeeding).

Advantages of Breastfeeding: Infant-related

- Less illness, less ear infections, less infections
- Less chance of obesity
- Bonding and needs met immediately
- Perfect nutrition and absorption rates
- Fewer allergies from antibodies
- Soothing and comforting for naps and getting back to sleep

How Long to Breastfeed?

Moms can produce milk as long as there is a need (it is all based on supply–demand once the baby is born). The American Academy of Pediatrics (AAP) recommends to breastfeed exclusively at least 6 months and to continue with additional solids at least one year (artificial formula would have to be used if breastfeeding stopped before one year). The WHO and LLL (La Leche League) recommend to breastfeed until the baby outgrows need (worldwide this occurs throughout toddlerhood). According to Katherine Dettwyler, author of *Breastfeeding: Biocultural Perspectives,* natural weaning occurs between ages of 2–6 years old. When weaning is a child-led concept, children not only benefit physiologically, but psychologically as well, leading to more happy and secure human beings. Breastfed babies are leaner for life—growth charts are different for breastfed babies—heavy for a few months then leaner.

How Long Should I Nurse My Baby?

Adapted from an article by Leaders of LLL of New York West

Breastfeeding is best-feeding. Nursing for even a day is the most precious gift you can give to your baby. How long should you nurse? These guidelines may help you to decide.

IF YOU NURSE FOR THE FIRST FEW DAYS, your baby will receive your colostrum, or early milk. Packed with optimal nutrition and antibodies, it helps get your baby's digestive system going and gives him his first—and easiest—"immunization." Breastfeeding gives your baby a great start and helps your own body recover from the birth, too. Taking time to relax and nurse is a lovely way to get to know your baby.

IF YOU NURSE FOR FOUR TO SIX WEEKS, you will ease the baby through the most critical part of infancy. Breastfed newborns are rarely sick or hospitalized and have few digestive problems. It takes four to six weeks to establish your milk supply and a good nursing relationship. Your body will recover naturally from childbirth. Remember—nursing mothers usually lose weight more easily! As an added bonus, prolactin, the "mothering hormone" that is produced every time you nurse, will help you and your baby form a special bond.

Advantages of Breastfeeding: Maternal-related

- Bonding and increased ability to sense baby's needs (hormonal response)
- Weight loss through caloric expenditure
- Convenient (no need for carrying feeding tools)
- Cost
- Decreases chance of uterine and breast cancer

IF YOU NURSE YOUR BABY FOR THREE OR FOUR MONTHS, you will do a great deal to avoid allergies, especially if they run in your family. The longer you wait before introducing other foods, the smaller the risk of allergic reactions.

IF YOU NURSE YOUR BABY FOR SIX MONTHS, you will supply all of your baby's nutritional needs for the first half year of her life. At this point, she may be ready to try some other foods. Nursing continues to ensure good health by providing antibodies to all the bacteria and viruses to which you or your baby are exposed. One study indicates that extended nursing reduces the risk of both childhood and some adult cancers.

IF YOU NURSE YOUR BABY FOR NINE MONTHS, you will see him through the fastest and most important development of his life on the most valuable of foods, your milk. Thanks to you, your baby is healthy, active, and alert, and the benefits of nursing for comfort and security become evident.

IF YOU NURSE YOUR BABY FOR A YEAR, you will have saved enough to buy a major appliance! Your baby is now ready to try a whole range of new foods. This year of nursing has given your child many health benefits that will last her whole life. She will have a stronger immune system, for example, and is less likely to need orthodontia or speech therapy. The American Academy of Pediatrics recommends: nursing for at least a year to ensure the best possible nutrition and health for your baby.

IF YOU NURSE YOUR BABY PAST A YEAR, you will continue to provide the highest quality nutrition and superb protection against illness at a time when infections are common. A toddler picks up everything! He is eating a variety of table foods and has had time to form a solid bond with you—a healthy starting point for his growing independence. Together you can work on the weaning process, progressing at a pace that he can handle. Former Surgeon General Antonia Novello has said, "It is the lucky baby . . . who continues to nurse until he's two."

IF YOU NURSE YOUR BABY UNTIL SHE OUTGROWS THE NEED, you can feel confident that you have met your baby's physical and emotional needs in the most natural and healthy way possible. In cultures where there is no pressure to wean, children tend to nurse for at least two years. The World Health Organization strongly encourages breastfeeding through toddlerhood. Your milk provides antibodies and other protective substances as long as you continue to nurse. Families of nursing toddlers often find that their medical bills are lower for years to come.

Children who were nursed long-term tend to be very secure. Nursing can help you both through the tears, tantrums, and tumbles of toddlerhood, while illnesses are milder and easier to handle. It is an all-purpose mothering tool that you won't want to be without! Don't worry that your child will nurse forever. All children eventually wean, no matter what you do. There are more nursing toddlers around than you might guess.

Some signs of an infant getting enough milk are

- Feeding the baby on cue (generally every 2 hours or sooner around the clock for 8–12 feeds per 24-hour period)
- 6 or more wet diapers a day
- Several stools a day in the first month
- Stools less firm and mustardy
- Infant is gaining weight and HAPPY
- Infant doubles weight in first 6 months and triples in one year

WHETHER YOU COUNT YOUR NURSING CAREER IN DAYS, WEEKS, MONTHS, OR YEARS, the decision to nurse your child is one that you will never regret. Weaning is a process, not an event. It is a big step for both of you, so let it take place gradually and with love.

Anatomy and Physiology of Breastfeeding

Changes in the breast occur throughout a female's life and especially during pregnancy to ready her for milk production. Those changes even begin when she is in utero herself. Two main hormones are involved with production and release of milk. **Prolactin** stimulates the production of milk, and **oxytocin** stimulates the release of milk from its storage cells and down through the ducts to the nipple (the "let-down reflex"). Human milk starts prenatally until about a few days postpartum as a substance called **colostrum**, the first milk, thick and yellowish in color, and high in proteins and antibodies, therefore antiinfectious factors. The **mature milk** "comes in" after 24–72 hours postpartum (quicker when mom and baby have drug-free labor and baby is able to breastfeed within an hour following birth). It is thinner and white/bluish in color and higher in calories and lower in protein.

Adding Foods to an Infant's Diet

The first solid foods start generally between 6–8 months when the baby sits up alone, opens mouth wide, and expresses interest. When offered before this time, allergies and malnutrition are more prevalent, and baby's intestines and enzymes are not ready (the starch enzyme amylase is not yet functioning). Babies will not be able to swallow solid foods and do best when they receive their nutrition from mom's milk exclusively the first half year. When the baby is able to start solids, offer brown rice cereal thinned with mom's milk with a soft spoon or your finger. Freshly pureed or smashed veggies and fruits such as avocados, cooked sweet potatoes, banana, and cooked carrots are popular first foods that babies love. Introduce proteins as they approach one year, preferably in the form of cooked lentils, black beans, and tofu, as these will not pose the food safety risks that eggs, poultry, and beef may pose. Oils and nut butters should not be introduced until into the second year, and any kind of hot dog, grapes, and popcorn may be choking hazards with infants and toddlers. Cow's milk may cause allergies, intestinal bleeding, excess protein overload on the kidneys, and Type I diabetes in infants, and honey may cause infant botulism. Avoid microwave use with infant food as it heats unevenly and may cause an injury to the infant. Microwaving breast milk also causes antibody damage.

Child Nutrition

Ellen Satter's "Division of Responsibility" is an excellent guideline for a healthy feeding relationship between the child and parent or caregiver.

Children seem to do well when offered nutritious choices and given the ability to choose how much to eat. They are actually better at eating intrinsically (for internal hunger and satiety reasons) whereas adults eat extrinsically (such as because they are tired, bored, lonely). The food pyramid or House may be used for children over 2 years of age, but serving sizes will be much smaller.

Parent's Role: Provide the choices, timing, and environment
Child's Role: Choose whether to eat and how much to eat

Get Kids Involved in the Kitchen

Meal pattern guidelines for ages 1–6 are listed in the following table. Keep in mind a 2-year-old may need to eat every 2 hours, eight times a day for his or her 1300 Calories per day (DRI). Snacks should be nutrient-dense because they will generally be the same amount of Calories as meals because the glycogen stores get filled, and they are unable to eat large adult-sized meals.

Meal Pattern Guidelines	Age 1 to 3	Age 4 to 6
Breakfast		
Mom's, cow or soy milk	1/2 cup	3/4 cup
Fruit	1/4 cup	1/4–1/2 cup
Whole-grain cereal or bread	1/3 ounce (1 Tbsp. per year) 1/2 slice	1/2 ounce (1 Tbsp. per year) 1/2–3/4 slice
Lunch		
Mom's, cow or soy milk	1/2 cup	3/4 cup
Protein group	1 ounce	1.5 ounces
Whole-grain bread, rice, or pasta	1/2 slice 1 Tbsp. per year	1/2–3/4 slice 1 Tbsp. per year
Vegetable or fruit	1/4 cup	1/4–1/2 cup
Dinner or Supper		
Mom's, cow or soy milk	1/2 cup	3/4 cup
Protein group	1 ounce	1.5 ounces
Whole-grain bread, rice, or pasta	1/2 slice 1 Tbsp. per year	1/2–3/4 slice 1 Tbsp. per year
Vegetable	1 Tbsp. per year	1 Tbsp. per year
Fruit	1/2 small fruit or 1 Tbsp. per year	1/2–3/4 small fruit or 1 Tbsp. per year
Snacks		
Mom's, cow, soy milk or yogurts or cheeses	1/4–1/2 cup 1/2-1 ounce	1/2 cup 1 ounce
Vegetable or fruit	1/4 cup	1/2 cup
Whole-grain bread, cereal, or other grains	1/2 slice 2 crackers 1/3 ounce	1/2–3/4 slice 2–3 crackers 1/2 ounce
Protein group	1/2 ounce	1/2 ounce

The Tbsp. per year refers to the age of the child (i.e., a 3-year-old needs three tablespoons).
"Protein" group examples are tofu, tempeh, beans, legumes, nuts, skinless poultry, and lean meat.

Great General Guidelines for Feeding Young Children

- One tablespoon per year (2 tablespoons of oatmeal is a serving for a 2-year-old)
- Number of years old is generally number of hours a child can go between meals for first 4–5 years (4-year-old may go 4 hours)
- Number of years old is generally the number of Calories plus 00 that a child can eat at one time for first 7–8 years (6-year-old can eat 600 Calories at one time)

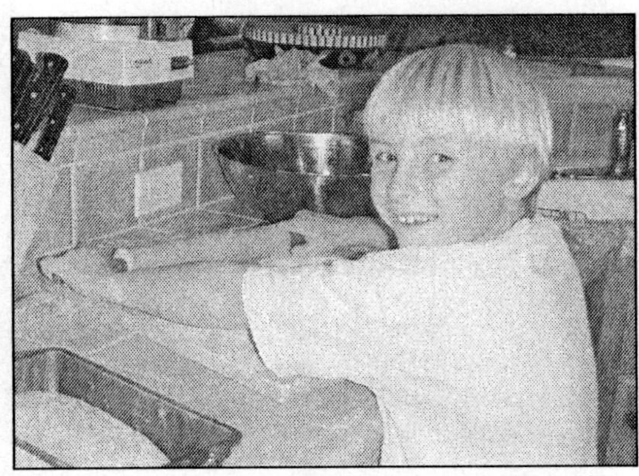
Get Kids Involved in the Kitchen

Some healthful tips for kid snacks are the following.

- Try to avoid hydrogenated and partially hydrogenated oils in products.
- Keep saturated fats low compared to unsaturated fats in foods.
- Avoid any fried foods.
- Choose almond butter over peanut butter when possible.
- Check sodium levels for excessiveness on labels (over 300–400 mg per serving).
- Try to avoid artificial additives and flavorings.
- Look for foods with less processed sugars like fruit juice and molasses than refined white sucrose (listed as "sugar").
- Keep simple sugar levels to less then 1/4–1/3 of total carbs (lower for "white" sugar).
- Choose whole-grain over white refined grain foods.
- Choose fresh fruits and veggies whenever possible.
- Pack two choices: possibly one from a fruit or veggie and one from the grain category.
- Choose purified water over concentrated juices for beverages.
- Choose organic whenever possible.
- Choose snacks with nutrient density as opposed to "empty calorie" sugar snacks.

The goal is: *Nutrient density/focus on "good fats"/complex unrefined carbs/some protein* (which will be in a healthful grain or bean snack naturally).

Some examples of these healthful snacks are as follows (remember to read food labels).

- Whole-grain crackers, pretzels, or breadsticks
- Popcorn
- Dry cereals (whole-grain like Shredded Spoonfuls and Puffins from TJ)
- Fresh fruit (apples, oranges, melon, pears, unsprayed strawberries, bananas, etc.)
- Fresh cut raw veggies with a healthful dip (carrots with hummus)
- Dried fruit (apricots, raisins, papaya)
- Yogurt with granolas
- Whole-grain muffins
- Raisins mixed with seeds or nuts
- Almond butter w/fruit jam on whole-wheat tortilla (2 together, then cut in triangles)
- Refried beans (low sodium, no lard) with baked tortilla chips (fresh guacamole also)
- If refrigeration is available, then low-fat dairy cheeses or soy cheeses on some of the above.

Healthful Snack Combinations for Anytime

Almond Butter Jam Torts
Homemade Applesauce

Refried Beans and Guacamole
Baked Tortilla Chips and Baby Carrots

Yummy Healthful Cereal Mix
Organic Strawberries/Banana Halves

Carrot-Raisin Muffins
Vanilla Soy Yogurt
Organic Granola

Creamy Peanut Butter on Sliced Apples
WW Thin Crackers

WW Bagel Bars
Baby Carrots/Hummus Dip

Watermelon Slices
Organic Popcorn
Nut/Dried Fruit Mix

Nutrition and Fitness for the Aging Population

The life expectancy in the United States is 73 years for men and 80 years for women. If you reach 80, you will more than likely live another 7–9 more years. Japan has the highest life expectancy (82 women, 76 men) and the 85+ group is the fastest growing segment in the United States. Currently 15% of the population is 65 years or older whom account for ~25% of all prescription medications used, ~40% of acute care hospital stays, and ~50% of the federal health budget. Of this group, 85% have nutrition-related problems.

What Is Aging?

Aging is the "processes of slow cell death" because cells age and die. The aging body can no longer keep up to replenish cells or meet demands. Aging may be caused by an error in copying the DNA that makes it no longer able to synthesize major protein, a stiffening of the connective tissue that decreases flexibility, alters organ function, and restrict nutrients from entering cells, more electron free radicals than the body can neutralize, a drop in the hormones, shrinking of the thymus gland and immune function, and that just cells are programmed to die and can only divide ~50 times. To increase life span and the quality of life some people decrease their energy intake with the belief of "Eat less and live longer," which has been named the Spartan diet. It is possible that eating less will cause less free radical damage and less cell turnover. Aerobic and strength-training exercise are healthful ways of increasing the number of possible cell divisions and avoiding free radical damage to the cells.

Physiological Function Decline with Aging

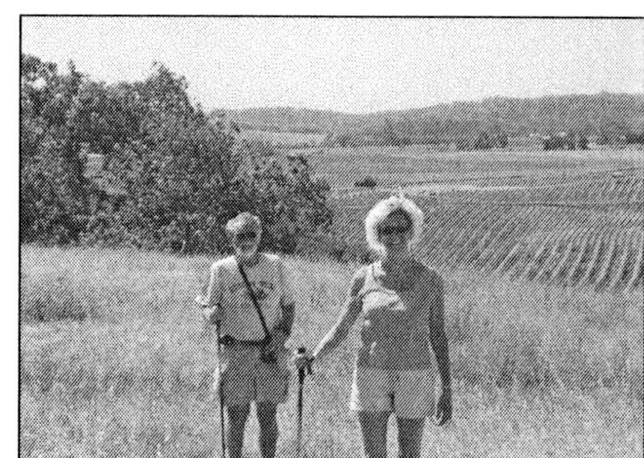

Hiking Keeps You Young in Your Sixties

There are many effects of aging such as decreased appetite, decreased sense of taste and smell, poor dental health, decrease sensation for thirst, constipation, decrease in lactase production, and less stomach acid production. Organ functions also decrease with age such as liver damage (associated with excess alcohol consumption), gallbladder problems such as gallstones from less bile production and decreased fat absorption, less insulin produced by the pancreas leading to high blood glucose, loss of nephrons in the kidneys leading decreased ability to excrete waste, decreased lung functioning, especially with smokers and people who don't exercise, decreased hearing and sight leading to less independence, a decrease in lean tissue from a shrinking of muscle cells, decreased basal metabolism, and increased fat stores. There is also a decline in cardiovascular health associated with a lack of physical activity, decline in cardiac output, and prevalence of heart attacks and strokes. Bone loss occurs leading to osteoporosis. Obesity is a result of overeating and lack of physical activity and contributes to high blood pressure and high blood glucose.

Slowing the Decline of Aging and Cell Damage

High carotenoids intake may help decrease retinal degeneration and an increase in physical activity and a low fat diet to decrease plaque formation is recommended. Monitor blood cholesterol, HDL, LDL, control blood pressure and meet the DRIs for vitamins B_6, B_{12} and folate.

Consume adequate calcium and vitamin D intake throughout life and participate in weight-bearing exercise for bone health (even at age 96, men and women can increase size and strength of muscle). Eat a moderate, but not high protein diet. New DRIs for seniors in the 51- to 70-year-old group and the > 70-year-old group reflect these recommendations, along with 2300 kcal for males; 1900 kcal for females, lower fat and sugar intake, lean proteins for zinc and vitamin B_6, six to eight cups of fluids a day, and high-fiber whole foods. Antioxidants can slow aging, HD, cataracts, arthritis, and cancer (ACE and selenium). Decrease fat to decrease arthritis symptoms. Because two-thirds of all elderly take prescriptions and these may interact with nutrients and affect appetite and may increase the loss of nutrients, extra amounts of these key nutrients may be needed.

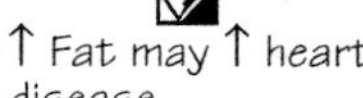

- ↑ Fat may ↑ heart disease
- ↑ Saturated fat may ↑ heart disease
- ↑ Hydrogenated fats may ↑ heart disease
- ↑ Phytochemicals may ↓ heart disease

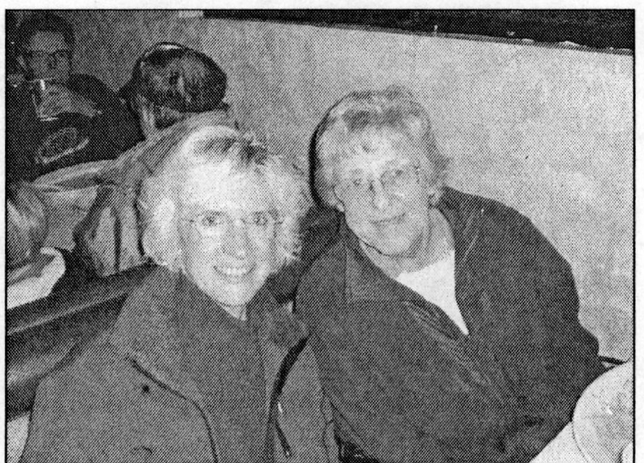
Sharing Mealtime Makes Good Nutrition Fun

The benefits of good nutrition choices will be delaying the onset of some diseases, improving your current condition, improving your quality of life, and more independence.

Community Nutrition Services

One-third of all elderly live in nursing homes and may be experiencing depression or loneliness from the loss of a loved one. Many need social support. There are community programs available to those aging adults that are less apt to prepare and cook their own meals such as meals-on-wheels, programs that provide lunch at a central location and provide one-third of the nutrient needs, federal commodity distribution, food stamps, and food cooperatives. Seek out these programs in your area and volunteer.

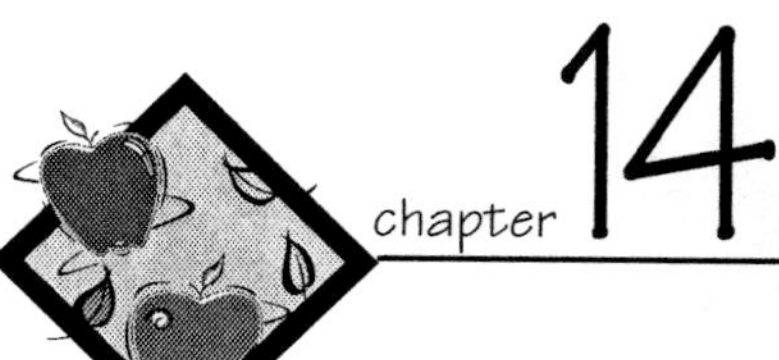

Consumer Nutrition— Putting It All Together

You have read all about the six categories of nutrients (carbohydrates, fats, proteins, vitamins, minerals, and water), and you are ready to apply your knowledge to planning, shopping, preparing, cooking, and enjoying your meals. This chapter takes you through these steps from planning to supermarket to consumption. Good luck in "Putting It All Together"!

Planning and Organizing Weekly Menus

An easy way to plan healthful varied meals is to use "The-Day-of-the-Week" plan and the "Three-Level Method of Meal Planning." Here are 10 easy steps to dinner planning:

Step 1 Decide what types of general dinners you like to eat and write them down.

Step 2 Categorize your meals according to a theme or the nation they come from. For example, use the categories Italian, Mexican, American, Cajun, etc.

Step 3 Decide how many nights per week you want to eat out (if any) and choose those nights.

Step 4 Write down the seven days of the week and match one category for each day. Remember to record your "eat out" days.

Step 5 Think of all the variations for each category.

Step 6 Label the variations 1, 2, or 3, depending on the length of preparation time. A short prep time of quick foods belong in Level 1. A medium prep time belongs in Level 2. A long "special occasion" prep time is a Level 3. Use your favorite cookbook recipes for level 3 meals.

Step 7 Complete your chart with the different level variations underneath each category.

Step 8 Shop for the ingredients and foods for a week.

Step 9 Post your chart someplace where you can see it. You will soon become so used to the meals and nightly themes that you will rarely need to look at the paper.

Step 10 Assign dinner prep to a responsible person in the house and make sure they know the plan! Enjoy!

50 Sample Dinner Plans using the "Nightly Theme" Method

C = Category or theme for that day of the week

1 = Level 1 (very quick prep)   2 = Level 2 (medium prep—author's favorite)   3 = Level 3 (recipe/longer prep)

All meals would include fresh raw (salad) and steamed (broccoli, carrots, etc.) vegetables.

Additional whole grains (brown rice, quinoa, couscous, etc.) added to many of the meals.

Sunday	**Monday**	**Tuesday**	**Wednesday**	**Thursday**	**Friday**	**Saturday**
C = Soup/Bread	***C = American w/ leftover soup***	***C = Mexican***	***C = Tempeh***	***C = Italian***	***C = Pizza***	***C = Stir-fry or Free Choice***
1 - Health Valley Quick Soups w/fresh veggies	1 - Boca Burgers w/lett, tom, avo on whole-grain bun	1 - Organic Refried Beans w/shredded soy cheese, TJ's guac, salsa, lett, tom on WW tort	1 - Ready-to-Eat Lemon Broil Tempeh Patties	1 - Any Shape Pasta w/Jar of Organic Marinara Sauce	1 - Delivered Veggie Pizza	1 - Restaurant: Big Sky
1 - Imagine Foods Quick Soups w/fresh veggies	1 - Tofu Dogs w/melted soy cheese and grilled onion on WW bun	1 - TJ's Frozen Organic Black Bean & Corn Enchiladas w/tom, guac	1 - Ready-to-Eat BBQ Tempeh Patties	1 - Any Shape Pasta w/premade pesto sauce	1 - Restaurant for Veggie Pizza	1 - Falafel on Pita
1 - Quick veget. chili from bulk or canned w/fresh veggies	1 - Garden Burgers w/lett, tom, avo on WW Sesame Bun	1 - TJ's Organic Bean Burritos w/tom, guac	2 - Tempeh Tacos w/veggies & warmed corn tortillas	1 - Olive oil w/baked tofu and soy cheese over noodles	1 - Frozen Amy's Soy Cheese Veggie Pizza	1 - Nonmeat Sloppy Joes
2 - Mixed Veggie Tofu Soup (veggies/tomato sauce/water/tofu)	2 - Grilled Portabello Mushroom & melted mozz. Soy cheese w/ lett, tom on WW Bun	2 - Black Bean Tamales w/Fresh Guac	2 - Tempeh Fajitas w/Multi-colored peppers	2 - Fresh Pesto Pasta (or Avocado Pesto) w/Polenta	2 - Homemade Toppings and Red Sauce on Thin-thin bread	2 - "Anything Goes" Stir-fry
2 - Homemade Lentil soup w/onions and carrots	2 - Marinated & Grilled Tofu w/lett, tom, avo on WW bun	2 - Bean and Rice or Quinoa Burritos w/lett, tom, home-made guac, salsa	2 - Stir-fried Tempeh Squares w/mixed veggies	2 - Homemade "Soy Cream Sauce" over Pasta	2 - Fresh Pesto on Thin-thin bread w/ fresh toppings	2 - Indian Curried Potato or Rice Dish
2 - Homemade Split Pea Soup w/Sweet Potatoes	3 - Homemade veggie bean burgers w/Works on WW	2 - Bean or Yves "nonmeat" hamburger tacos	2 - Tempeh-Veggie Shish Kabobs	2 - Mushroom Sauce Noodle Casserole	3 - Homemade Crust AND Toppings	2 - Vegetarian Sushi
2 - Homemade Black bean Chili w/veggies		3 - Bean, Rice, Corn Casserole		3 - Homemade Tofu Manicotti		3 - Spinach Tofu Quiche
2 - Homemade Mixed Bean Soup w/veggies		3 - Homemade Tamales		3 - Homemade Spinach Tofu Lasagna		3 - Homemade dish from favorite cookbook

Shopping for Healthful Foods and Reading Food Labels

Supermarkets can be overwhelming and chock full of refined, hydrogenated, low-nutrient dense, sugary choices. A first step in supermarket shopping is to choose those stores that have healthful options such as natural food cooperatives in your area or healthful chains such as Whole Foods Market. To evaluate the food, be sure to look at the label to decide if the food fits into your nutritional plan (non-hydrogenated/only 1/4–1/3 sugar for cereals, etc.).

Review the anatomy of a food label and descriptive terms for label reading to help you learn more about label reading.

Anatomy of a Food Label

The sample shown, provided by the Food and Drug Administration, is for boxed macaroni and cheese.

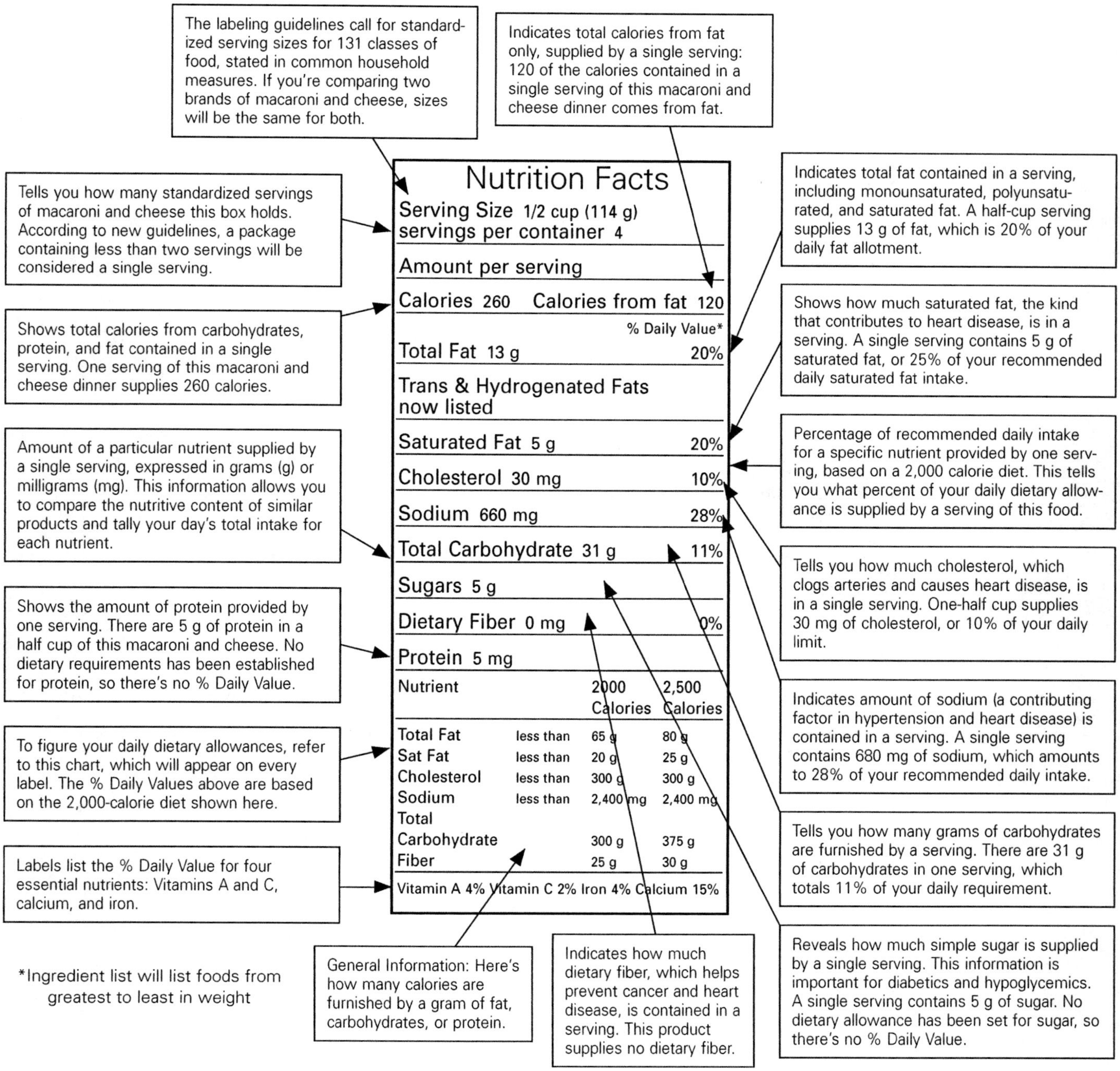

Nutrition Facts

Serving Size 1/2 cup (114 g)
servings per container 4

Amount per serving

Calories 260 Calories from fat 120

	% Daily Value*
Total Fat 13 g	20%
Trans & Hydrogenated Fats now listed	
Saturated Fat 5 g	20%
Cholesterol 30 mg	10%
Sodium 660 mg	28%
Total Carbohydrate 31 g	11%
Sugars 5 g	
Dietary Fiber 0 mg	0%
Protein 5 mg	

Nutrient		2000 Calories	2,500 Calories
Total Fat	less than	65 g	80 g
Sat Fat	less than	20 g	25 g
Cholesterol	less than	300 g	300 g
Sodium	less than	2,400 mg	2,400 mg
Total Carbohydrate		300 g	375 g
Fiber		25 g	30 g

Vitamin A 4% Vitamin C 2% Iron 4% Calcium 15%

The labeling guidelines call for standardized serving sizes for 131 classes of food, stated in common household measures. If you're comparing two brands of macaroni and cheese, sizes will be the same for both.

Indicates total calories from fat only, supplied by a single serving: 120 of the calories contained in a single serving of this macaroni and cheese dinner comes from fat.

Tells you how many standardized servings of macaroni and cheese this box holds. According to new guidelines, a package containing less than two servings will be considered a single serving.

Shows total calories from carbohydrates, protein, and fat contained in a single serving. One serving of this macaroni and cheese dinner supplies 260 calories.

Amount of a particular nutrient supplied by a single serving, expressed in grams (g) or milligrams (mg). This information allows you to compare the nutritive content of similar products and tally your day's total intake for each nutrient.

Shows the amount of protein provided by one serving. There are 5 g of protein in a half cup of this macaroni and cheese. No dietary requirements has been established for protein, so there's no % Daily Value.

To figure your daily dietary allowances, refer to this chart, which will appear on every label. The % Daily Values above are based on the 2,000-calorie diet shown here.

Labels list the % Daily Value for four essential nutrients: Vitamins A and C, calcium, and iron.

Indicates total fat contained in a serving, including monounsaturated, polyunsaturated, and saturated fat. A half-cup serving supplies 13 g of fat, which is 20% of your daily fat allotment.

Shows how much saturated fat, the kind that contributes to heart disease, is in a serving. A single serving contains 5 g of saturated fat, or 25% of your recommended daily saturated fat intake.

Percentage of recommended daily intake for a specific nutrient provided by one serving, based on a 2,000 calorie diet. This tells you what percent of your daily dietary allowance is supplied by a serving of this food.

Tells you how much cholesterol, which clogs arteries and causes heart disease, is in a single serving. One-half cup supplies 30 mg of cholesterol, or 10% of your daily limit.

Indicates amount of sodium (a contributing factor in hypertension and heart disease) is contained in a serving. A single serving contains 680 mg of sodium, which amounts to 28% of your recommended daily intake.

Tells you how many grams of carbohydrates are furnished by a serving. There are 31 g of carbohydrates in one serving, which totals 11% of your daily requirement.

General Information: Here's how many calories are furnished by a gram of fat, carbohydrates, or protein.

Indicates how much dietary fiber, which helps prevent cancer and heart disease, is contained in a serving. This product supplies no dietary fiber.

Reveals how much simple sugar is supplied by a single serving. This information is important for diabetics and hypoglycemics. A single serving contains 5 g of sugar. No dietary allowance has been set for sugar, so there's no % Daily Value.

*Ingredient list will list foods from greatest to least in weight

Descriptive Terms Used on Food Labels

Energy Terms

low calorie: 40 calories or fewer per serving.
reduced calorie: at least 25% lower in calories than a "regular," or reference, food.
calorie free: fewer than 5 calories per serving.

Fat Terms (Meat and Poultry Products)

extra lean
less than 5 g of fat *and*
less than 2 g of saturated fat *and*
less than 95 mg of cholesterol per serving.
lean
less than 10 g of fat *and*
less than 4 g of saturated fat *and*
less than 95 mg of cholesterol per serving.

Fat and Cholesterol Terms (All Products)

cholesterol free
less than 2 mg cholesterol *and*
2 g or less saturated fat per serving.
fat free: less than 0.5 g of fat per serving.
low cholesterol
20 mg or less of cholesterol *and*
2 g or less saturated fat per serving.
low fat: 3 g or less fat per serving.
low saturated fat: 1 g or less saturated fat per serving.
percent fat free may be used only if the product meets the definition of *low fat* or *fat free*. Requires disclosure of g fat per 100 g food.
reduced or less cholesterol
at least 25% less cholesterol than a reference food *and*
2 g or less saturated fat per serving.
reduced saturated fat
25% or less of saturated fat *and*
reduced by more than 1 g saturated fat per serving compared with a reference food.
saturated fat free
less than 0.5 g of saturated fat *and*
less than 0.5 g of *trans*-fatty acids.

Fiber Terms

high fiber: 5 g or more per serving. (Foods making high-fiber claims must fit the definition of low fat, or the level of total fat must appear next to the high-fiber claim.)
good source of fiber: 2.5 g to 4.9 g per serving.
more or **added fiber:** at least 2.5 g more per serving than a reference food.

Other Terms

free, without, no, zero, none or a trivial amount: *Calorie free* means containing fewer than 5 calories per serving; *sugar free or fat free* means containing less than half a gram per serving.
fresh: raw, unprocessed, or minimally processed with no added preservatives.
good source: 10 to 19% of the Daily Value per serving.
healthy: low in fat, saturated fat, cholesterol, and sodium and containing at least 10% of the Daily Value for vitamin A, vitamin C, iron, calcium, protein, or fiber.
high in: 20% or more of the Daily Value for a given nutrient per serving; synonyms include "rich in" or "excellent source."
less, fewer, reduced: containing at least 25% less of a nutrient or calories than a reference food. This may occur naturally or as a result of altering the food. For example, pretzels, which are usually low in fat, can claim to provide less fat than potato chips, a comparable food.
light: this descriptor has three meanings on labels:
1. A serving provides one-third fewer calories or half the fat of the regular product.
2. A serving of a low-calorie, low-fat food provides half the sodium normally present.
3. The product is light in color and texture, so long as the label makes this intent clear, as in "light brown sugar."

more, extra: at least 10% more of the Daily Value than in a reference food. The nutrient may be added or may occur naturally.

Sodium Terms

low sodium: 140 mg or less sodium per serving.
sodium free: less than 5 mg per serving.
very low sodium: 35 mg or less per serving.

 Healthful Sample Shopping Check Sheet (try to choose organic)

General Food	***Subcategory***	***Subcategory***	***Subcategory***	***Subcategory***
Whole Grains	**Whole Bulk Grains** ♦ Barley ♦ Brown rice ♦ Amaranth ♦ Buckwheat ♦ Cornmeal ♦ Popcorn ♦ Rye triticle ♦ Quinoa ♦ Millet ♦ 9-grain cereals ♦ Oats ♦ Wholesome granolas ♦ Hot cereal grains ♦ Whole grain flours ♦ Whole grain pastas	**Whole-Grain Cereals** ♦ Shredded wheat ♦ Whole O's ♦ Puffed rice, corn, millet, wheat ♦ Healthful granola ♦ Bran flakes ♦ Most "Barbara's" cereal ♦ Many TJ* ♦ Most "Kashi" ♦ Most "Health Valley" ♦ Most "Nature's Path" ♦ Cream of rye ♦ Cream of rice	**Whole-Grain (look for "whole" before the grain) Breads** ♦ Tortilla ♦ Corn tortilla ♦ Pita ♦ Sprouted grain bread ♦ Bagels ♦ Muffins ♦ Thin bread for wraps ♦ Chapatti ♦ Burger buns ♦ Dog buns ♦ English muffins ♦ Fresh loaves	**Quick Whole Grains** ♦ Soba noodles ♦ Westbrae ramen ♦ Fantastic Food mixes ♦ Arrowhead Mill mixes ♦ Lundberg mixes ♦ Brown rice milk ♦ Brown rice cakes ♦ Crackers
Veggies & Fruits	**Whole Local Fresh Veggies from Farmer's Market, Food Co-op, or Community Garden** ♦ Broccoli ♦ Cauliflower ♦ Leafy greens (kale, bok choy, mustard, chard) ♦ Mushroom ♦ Yellow and purple onion ♦ Squash ♦ R/Y/G bell peppers ♦ Carrot ♦ Tomato ♦ Sea vegetables	**Whole Local Fresh Fruits from Farmer's Market, Food Co-op, or Garden** ♦ Papaya ♦ Mango ♦ Melon ♦ Banana ♦ Strawberries ♦ Blueberries ♦ Grapes ♦ Kiwi ♦ Apple ♦ Orange ♦ Grapefruit	**Dried Fruits and Veggies** ♦ Figs ♦ Dates ♦ Raisins ♦ Apricot ♦ Apples ♦ Prunes ♦ Papaya ♦ Pineapple ♦ Banana ♦ Peas ♦ Corn ♦ Blueberries ♦ Cranberries	**Fruit and Veggie Products** ♦ 100% fruit juice ♦ 100% fruit jam ♦ Veggie chips ♦ 100% fruit roll-ups ♦ Veggie burgers ♦ Marinara sauce
Protein Sources	**Whole Beans and Legumes** ♦ Garbanzo beans ♦ Adzuki beans ♦ Black-eyed peas ♦ Split-peas ♦ Red and green lentils ♦ Black, red, small white, and kidney beans ♦ Soy bean ♦ Pinto beans ♦ Lima beans ♦ Whole green peas	**Quick Legumes** ♦ "Eden Foods" canned ♦ Most TJ canned (organic) ♦ "Fantastic Foods" beans and soups ♦ "Health Valley" beans and soups	**Soy Products** ♦ Soy dogs (Yves) ♦ Soy cheese (TofuRella) ♦ Soy yogurt (Silk) ♦ Soy milk (TJ and Silk) ♦ Tempeh burgers ♦ Tofu ♦ Soy deli slices (Yves) ♦ Soy ground round ♦ Soy parmesan	**Frozen Meals** ♦ Amy's Enchiladas ♦ Amy's Pockets ♦ Amy's Burritos ♦ Amy's Bowls ♦ Amy's Pot Pies ♦ Amy's Pizza ♦ Amy's Soups ♦ Amy's Veggie Burgers ♦ TJ Burritos ♦ TJ Enchiladas

*TJ=Trader Joe's

(continued)

Healthful Sample Shopping Check Sheet (continued)

General Food	Subcategory	Subcategory	Subcategory	Subcategory
Condiments	**Fresh and Raw Nuts and Seeds** ◆ Walnuts ◆ Almonds ◆ Cashews ◆ Brazil nuts ◆ Pecans ◆ Nut butters ◆ Flax seed ◆ Sunflower seed ◆ Sesame seed	**Oils and Margarines** ◆ Canola ◆ Olive ◆ Safflower ◆ Nonhydrogenated Canola Margarine (Spectrum Naturals)	**Spreads and Dips** ◆ Ketchup ◆ Mustard ◆ Nayonaise (NaSoya) ◆ Salsa ◆ Fresh guacamole ◆ Hummus	**Salad Dressings** ◆ Nasoya brands ◆ Seeds of Change brand ◆ TJ* Italian brand ◆ Simply Delicious brand
More Snacks & Desserts	**"Ice Cream"/Bars/ Sandwiches** ◆ Soy Delicious brand ◆ Soy Dream brand ◆ Rice Dream brand	**"Chips"** ◆ Baked "Kettle" brand ◆ Baked "Guiltless Gourmet" brand	**Pastry Poppers** ◆ Amy's Frozen ◆ Nature's Path ◆ Nature's Warehouse	**Energy Bars & Cookies** ◆ Clif ◆ Powerbar ◆ Shady Maple Farms ◆ TJ* Oatmeal/ch chip
Beverages	**Water** ◆ Arrowhead ◆ Calistoga Sparkling ◆ Perrier ◆ Pellengrino	**Herbal Tea & Grain "Coffee"** ◆ Celestial Seasonings ◆ Traditional Medicinals ◆ Postum ◆ Roma		

*TJ=Trader Joe's

Another way to look at dietary choices (other than the Healthful House of Food) is to look at foods in order from best to worst in terms of overall nutrition, nutrient density, and phytochemicals.

The Most Nutritious Food Choices with Examples—Based on Nutrient Density, Overall Nutrition, and Disease-Fighting Properties

Food	In order The BEST and EAT THE MOST....to FOODS to EAT THE LEAST	Cherie's Ranking of Foods According to Quality (choose foods from the top the most; the bottom the least)
Organic dark greens (kale, chard, bok choy, seaweed, collard greens)		1
Organic cruciferous vegetables (carrot, broccoli, cauliflower, brussels sprouts)		2
Organic whole grains (brown rice, millet, barley, kamut, quinoa, oats)		3
Organic fresh vegetable juices (carrot, spinach, parsley, celery, beet, garlic)		4
Organic other whole vegetables (onion, yellow squash, red pepper, sweet potato, potato, tomato)		5
Organic whole and sprouted beans (black beans, split peas, lentils, pintos, soy beans)		6
Organic legume and bean products (tempeh, tofu, black bean dip, soy milk, soy cheese, soy yogurt)		7
Organic whole fruits (papaya, mango, melon, grapefruit, strawberry, orange, apple)		8
Organic whole-grain products (bread, pasta, crackers, muffins, bagels)		9
Organic whole nuts and seeds (almonds, walnuts, flax, cashew, sunflower, sesame)		10
Organic oils (olive, canola, safflower, nonhydrogenated and low saturated fat canola margarines)		11
Reduced-fat dairy (cheese, yogurt, milk)		12
Fish, turkey, and chicken		13
Coffee, soda, alcohol, and refined sugar snacks		14
Deep sea animals, whole fat dairy and eggs, butter, red meat, and pork		15

Preparing Healthful Foods in the Home

Most people are used to the grain wheat, but many other nutritious whole grains are available. The following is a listing of several grains and their descriptions:

Grain Descriptions

Barley

This grain grinds into a very fine, white flour that can be used to make white gravies and to vary whole-grain breads. It is high in malt and has a delightful, mild flavor.

Buckwheat

This seed is not actually one of the grains, but because of its chemical content is widely used in the same fashion that grains are used. It has a fairly strong flavor, and when used whole or as the flour, it is well to mix it with one of the more bland grains such as corn, rice, or millet. It has a high biologic value, being rich in vitamins and minerals; it deserves much greater popularity than just as buckwheat pancakes.

Corn

Corn was first grown in North America and continues to be our most widely used grain in this hemisphere. Being a large grain on a large ear, it grows well and is an important seed crop. When used in rotation with the other grains, it is an important nutrient. It should be considered, as with all the grains, to be one among many, and not a steady diet. Corn can be used in the "milk stage" as whole kernel or cream corn, and served as a vegetable in the menu. It has many uses as the hoecake, griddle cake, waffle, mixed with soybean flour to make a raised cornbread, chapitis, fritos, enchiladas, and tortillas. By using a coarse grind, grits are produced that can be used in a variety of ways: (1) breakfast porridge, (2) congealed porridge sliced and baked, or (3) mixed with other grains. Serving grits and gravy, use a variety of fruit sauces, numerous nut or soy spreads such as peanut butter or almond-date jam, no-oil mayonnaise, tomato gravy, etc.

Millet

Millet is a cereal commonly used in Europe and gaining much popularity in this hemisphere. It has a bland flavor and can be used in much the same way as corn or rice.

Oats

This is one of our more common cereal grains of quite high biologic value. It can be used as the whole grain, the rolled grain, grits or coarse cracked oats, flour or meal. The flours can be used in breads, and the other forms can be cooked as breakfast foods, or used to give body to casserole dishes and stews, and to make patties or burgers. This important grain has many uses and should not be thought of merely as "oatmeal." Try oatburgers.

Rice

The most important grain in the economy of the orient, rice has kept much of China alive and healthy for the last three centuries. Not until polishing the grain became a common practice did nutritional deficiencies exist in China when rice was abundant. It has a very high quality protein and many essential vitamins and minerals. One who is on a varied diet of fruits and vegetables will have his diet completed by rice. The great travesty against this grain is polishing. Use brown rice.

Rye

This hardy cereal grain is widely grown for its grain as well as its straw. It makes a quick-growing pasture grass in some of its species. The flour made from rye should be used to vary the nutritive content of breads, to make gravies, and to thicken soups and casserole dishes. Very delightful breakfast cereals can be made by using several kinds of grains together.

Wheat

There are many grains in this group of cereal grasses. Each of the different species has somewhat different amino acid content as well as vitamin and mineral spectrum. Generally, when bread is spoken of, one thinks of wheat bread. Like rice, it has been subjected to a great injustice in that the major nutritive properties are removed in the milling process for the production of a finer flour and a product that will keep for long periods on the grocery shelf. The long keeping quality of white flour is due to the separation of the rich vitamin and mineral bearing oils, which are likely to become rancid. Bugs do not so readily attack the white flour products because the bugs recognize that the product is inferior and will not support their lives.

Breakfast: Start the Day Right!

Breakfast can be a special time for families to begin their day together. Proper nutrition can be made simple by using a variety of natural foods. Try using a different grain each morning of the week to provide an interesting and balanced menu.

Cooking Time Chart for Cereals and Grains

Grain (1 cup)	Water (in cups)	Time (in minutes)
Barley, hulled, not pearled	3	60
rolled	2–3	30–45
Buckwheat groats	2	20
Cornmeal	4	45–60
Millet, hulled	3	45–60
Oats, whole	4–5	2–3 hours
rolled (oatmeal)	2–3	30–45
Rice, brown (fluffy)	2	45–50
(creamy)	4	60
cream of rice (flour)	4	30
Rye berries	4–5	2 hours
flaked	2	30–45
Wheat berries	4–5	3 hours
cream of wheat	3	30
cracked wheat	3	30–40
flaked	2	30–45

The amount of water often depends on whether you enjoy your cereal thick or gruel style

Quick Nutritious Balanced Breakfast Choices

Many of our active lifestyles do not allow time to cook hot grains, so the following lists several quick choices for a healthful breakfast. The following choices are low in fat (10%–15%), high in complex carbohydrates and fiber, and ~200–250 calories each. (Combine two or double if you are active.)

1. Hot Cereal (oatmeal, cream of rye, cream of rice, etc.)
   - ¼–⅓ cup dry
   - Add one serving of fruit for sweetener (banana or ¼ cup raisins or 1 cup strawberries, etc.)
   - Use 1 tbsp. apple juice or honey or pure maple syrup if desired
2. Cold Cereal (whole grain choices without sugar)
   - 200 calorie serving (= ½ cup for granola, = 1 cup flake, = 2 cups puffed)
   - Add one piece of fruit for sweetener or buy fruit-sweetened cereals (Health Valley, Barbara's, Nature's Path, Erewhon, etc.)
   - Use ½ cup soy, brown rice, or nonfat or 1% cow's milk
3. Muffin (whole grain carrot, apple, or zucchini)
4. Bagels (Preferably whole grain water bagels)
   - Spread nonsweetened jams or fresh fruit
   - Sesame, Apple Walnut, Regular
   - Whole Wheat, Cinnamon Raisin, Poppyseed
   - Spread with nut butters in moderation (almond or soy more nutrient dense)
5. Toast (whole grain)
   - Spread nonsweetened jams or fresh fruit and/or nut butter
6. Fresh Fruit (banana, papaya, strawberries, apples, etc.)
7. Pancakes or Waffles (Preferably some type of whole grain)
   - Add fruit for sweetener or pure maple syrup
   - Use nonhydrogenated margarine or almond butter
8. Fresh Fruit Smoothie
   - Visit your local smoothie shop
   - Make your own by mixing in blender:

     ice
     1 banana
     1 tablespoon fresh nut butter or 3 oz. tofu
     ¼ cup apple juice, rice milk, or soy milk
     ½ cup strawberries

Some Fun Additional Breakfast Ideas

- Red potatoes sauteed in a little canola oil with onions and peppers.
- Breakfast burritos with mashed pinto beans, chopped chilies, chopped tomato, and chopped cilantro wrapped in a whole wheat tortilla.
- Add low-fat plain yogurt or soy yogurt to the meal.
- Breakfast burritos with tempeh or tofu in place of the beans.
- Top off breakfast with 4 oz. of calcium-fortified grapefruit juice!

Sample Breakfast

2 medium bowls of shredded spoonfuls and granola with banana, strawberries, rice milk, and a cup of grapefruit juice = ~173 grams of wholesome carbohydrates!

Sample Carbohydrate Grams of Breakfast Options

¾ cup Shredded Spoonfuls	24 grams
½ cup Granola	34 grams
1 cup Frosted Wheat	44 grams
Bagel	64 grams
Toast	22 grams
Banana	28 grams
½ cup strawberries	15 grams
Rice milk	26 grams
Soy milk	17 grams
Grapefruit juice	22 grams
Yogurt	24 grams
1 Tbsp. jam	6 grams

Preparing Vegetables

Best Methods for Cooking Vegetables

1. Cook without water, if possible.
2. Cook as short a time as possible and just before serving.
3. Avoid bruising, soaking, or wilting vegetables.

4. Keep vegetables cold until ready to cook.
5. Buy organic or pesticide-free whenever possible.
6. Do not remove cover while cooking.
7. Avoid the use of utensils that are chipped, worn, have copper alloys or are made of aluminum.
8. Use plastic scouring pad or stiff brush for vegetables. A stainless steel metal mesh pad may be used but be sure to check vegetables for tiny pieces that could cling to them.
9. When done, vegetables should have a crisp, tender texture. Overcooked they are mush, strong flavored and lose attractive natural color.
10. Cook vegetables whole or in large pieces when possible. Cook with skins on to save nutrients. Be sure potatoes have all green removed and thick patches of skin.
11. Lightly steam veggies to retain nutritive value.
12. A small amount of lemon juice added to the cooking water will help restore the color of red cabbage and beets.
13. Serve as soon as the vegetable is cooked. Keeping vegetables warm after they are cooked causes loss of food value, particularly vitamins. If they must wait, allow to cool, then reheat.

Seasoning Vegetables

There are many ways to make vegetables taste well seasoned without using too much salt.

Herbs can be used to enhance the natural flavors of foods. There are no rules to seasoning. Experiment. If you are unfamiliar with an herb, try its effect on various foods by using a small amount at first. If the flavor needs to blend in certain foods, add the flavor at the beginning. If the flavor is to be kept distinct from the food it is used with, add just before serving. Long cooking destroys flavor. Fresh herbs are more desirable in salads. Use three times as much fresh than if dried.

The use of lemon juice can perk up the food. Tomato can be used in a similar way, raw and chopped, canned, as sauce or puree. Onion, green pepper, celery, parsley, or garlic will add interesting touches. The addition of chopped nuts or seeds, such as sesame, add a delightful flavor.

Suggested Seasonings

Asparagus: Lemon juice, Golden sauce, slivered almonds
Beets: Tarragon, sweet basil, thyme, bay leaf, lemon juice
Broccoli: Tarragon, marjoram, oregano, lemon juice, sesame seeds, Cashew-Pimiento Cheese Spread
Brussels Sprouts: Sweet basil, dill, savory, thyme
Carrots: Sweet basil, dill, thyme, marjoram, parsley, mint, onion rings, cream sauce
Cauliflower: Rosemary, savory, dill, Cashew-Pimiento Cheese Spread, parsley, paprika
Cabbage: Caraway, celery seed, savory, dill
Corn: Dill, sweet basil, pimiento, parsley, green pepper
Cucumbers: Tarragon, sweet basil, savory, dill, lemon juice, paprika
Eggplant: Sweet basil, thyme, oregano, sage, tomato
Beans (dried): Sweet basil, oregano, dill, savory, cumin, garlic, parsley, bay leaf, tomato
Green Beans: Sweet basil, dill, thyme, marjoram, oregano, savory, tomato, onion, garlic, almonds, mushrooms
Lima Beans: Sweet basil, chives, savory
Onions: Oregano, thyme, sweet basil
Peas: Sweet basil, mint, savory, oregano, dill, mushrooms, parsley
Potatoes: Dill, chives, sweet basil, marjoram, savory, parsley
Squash: Sweet basil, dill, oregano, savory, flake yeast
Spinach: Tarragon, thyme, oregano, rosemary
Tomatoes: Sweet basil, oregano, marjoram, onion, garlic, sage
Green Salad Dressing: Sweet basil, oregano, marjoram, onion, garlic, sage
Chili Substitute: Spanish onions with cumin

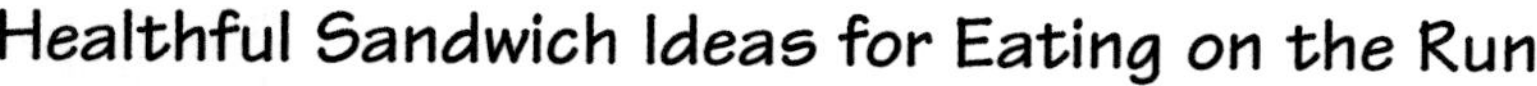

Healthful Sandwich Ideas for Eating on the Run

The average American eats not only too much fat, but too much protein in his/her daily diet. The following is a list of lunchtime or anytime sandwich suggestions to substitute for the "Americanized" lunch of high-fat and high-protein beef, pork, cold cuts, hamburgers, fish, and tuna. Experiment with different foods and enjoy!

1. Tofu Salad: (NaSoya Mayo, Tofu, Carrots, Cucumber, Vegit Seasoning, Tumeric—mix in food processor) on whole grain bread with mustard and sprouts.
2. Tempeh Burgers: Good brands are already seasoned—Light Life and White Wave. Cook in a skillet 3–5 minutes with a little water or canola oil spray to keep from sticking and then prepare on toasted whole-grain bun, bread, or pita with veggies and condiments of choice. (Examples—dark green lettuce, tomato, onion, sprouts, honey-sweetened ketchup, mustard, "nayonaise"). This is a terrific sandwich packed with vitamins, minerals, fiber, complex carbohydrates, and protein.
3. Veggie Combo: Whole-grain bread, bun, or pita with the veggies and condiments of your choice. (Example—avocado slices, tomato, sprouts, mustard, and "nayonaise").
4. Sesame, Tofu, Nature Burger: Whole-grain bread, bun, or pita with veggies and condiments of choice. Quick-mix packages make these simple and tasty!
5. Soy Cheese/Avocado: Serve on whole-grain type bread and add more veggies and condiments of your choice.
6. Healthful "Cold Cuts": Turkey and beef-flavored products for the person who loves the taste of these products, but does not desire the unhealthful ingredients with the traditional cold cuts. "Phoney Baloney" deli slices from Yves are available. Serve on whole-grain bread with sprouts and mustard.
7. Almond, Cashew, or Peanut Butter/Unsweetened Jam or Fresh Fruit (sliced strawberries or bananas): Nut butters are high in fat, but not animal fat, therefore they contain no cholesterol and supply healthful fats. They still should be used sparingly for those trying to lose body fat and reduce their total dietary fat.

Easy Dinner Ideas

1. Pastas (Italian Theme)
    - Preferably whole-grain, corn, soy, or another less-refined grain
    - Top with any steamed or lightly stir-fried veggies you prefer
        - Marinara or tomato-based sauce
        - Avocado pesto or olive oil/pine nut/garlic
            - Lemon juice, cilantro, avocado, garlic
            - Serve with red potatoes and green beans mixed in
        - Use "soyco" parmesan or nutritional yeast for topping or sauce
        - Use healthful dressings as sauces
        - Vary serving pastas both hot and cold
        - Try varying veggies—onions, squash, mushrooms, zucchini, tomato, kale, bok choy, etc.
        - Vary noodle shape, size, and type (try soba, ramen, etc.)
2. Burritos/Wraps (Mexican Theme)
    - Use whole-grain flour (no lard) or corn tortillas (hint: best when cooked straight off the stove burner and browned) or thin bread
    - Stuff with any combo of veggies (avocado slices, tomato, mushrooms, shredded carrots, baked zucchini, etc.)
    - Use different types of beans (black, kidney, pinto, etc.)
    - Alternate homemade, and canned low-fat w/canola oil beans
    - If cheese is desired, try different varieties of soy cheese or low-fat cheese
    - Dressing includes salsas or salad dressings, depending on if beans were used

- Also include a grain if desired—barley, brown rice, etc.
- Use grilled or baked tofu or tempeh for burritos or tacos
- Make your own salsa in a food processor with garlic, onion, lemon juice, cilantro, Jalapeño pepper, and tomato (put tomato in last to lightly chop)

3. GRAIN/VEGGIE MEALS
   - Cook any grain
   - Cook combo of fresh veggies in a wok starting with a little water or olive or canola oil and garlic and onions, then adding firmest veggies next, and softest last
   - Good wok veggies are green peppers, Chinese cabbage, snow peas, green beans, broccoli, kale, bok choy, zucchini, squash, carrots, etc.
   - Stir-fry mixture together and season with herbs or combo seasonings
   - Tofu, baked tofu, and tempeh may also be included

4. SOUPS, SUSHI, AND MORE!
   - Serve soups with crackers or bread and a salad for a complete meal
   - Try a variety of soups—split pea, lentil, bean, veggie, mushroom, barley, etc.
   - Serve homemade chili or dried (add water) or canned Health Valley over rice
   - "The Food Merchant's Brand" Polenta is yummy and only requires slicing and heating
   - Sushi wraps are almost as quick as burritos—avocado, mango, sunflower sprouts, and cucumber slices rolled up with brown rice in nori
   - Tempeh tacos are a favorite
   - Super salads
   - Potatoes—mashed, baked, broiled, sliced and baked as fries
   - Spinach-Tofu Quiche

5. "AMERICAN" THEME ALTERNATIVES
   - Choose one of the many veggie, grain, mushroom or tempeh burgers (Boca Burgers, Garden Burgers, Okra Burgers)
   - Serve with "nayonaise" by NaSoya, mustard, sprouts, lettuce, and tomato
   - Serve open-faced or on a whole grain bun or bread
   - Veggie dogs on whole wheat bun *or* wrapped in a whole wheat tortilla with TJ Vegetarian Chili and shredded cheese (author's camping favorite).

Build a Super Salad

Pat Brown, M.S., R.D., *Cuesta College. Reprinted by permission.*

A crisp salad full of fresh vegetables is a great complement to soup or pasta, or it can be a meal by itself with a good loaf of bread. Here are some ideas to get you started building your own super salads.

- **Lettuce** Avoid iceberg lettuce, it's extremely low in nutrients. The bags of salad "mixes" are certainly convenient, but they're also expensive, and the cut up leaves will lose some nutrients. Choose romaine to get the lettuce with the highest nutrient content. The darker the green color of a lettuce, the more nutrients it will contain.

  The following method will provide you with prewashed greens that will keep a week in the refrigerator with minimal nutrient loss. Take a head of romaine and slice off the bottom 3 inches. This should separate the leaves so that they can be submerged in a sinkfull of water. Swish the leaves around to remove any dirt. Spin the leaves dry in a salad spinner if you have one, or place the greens on a kitchen towel, pick up the four corners and swing it around to remove excess water. If they're really wet, you may wish to do your swinging outside. You will need a 1-gallon size, zippered-type plastic bag and two sheets of paper towels to store the lettuce. Place one paper towel flat in the plastic bag. Select the shorter inner leaves of the head and place them in the bottom of the bag, followed by the outer leaves. Then slide the second paper towel over the leaves so that they are sandwiched between the two layers of paper toweling. Zip up the bag and refrigerate. Then when you want to make a salad, take out as many leaves as you'll need and tear them up into your salad bowl.

- **Vegetables** The best vegetables to include in your salad are those that provide plenty of vitamins, minerals, fiber, antioxidants, and phytochemicals. Select six or more from the following.

Carrots	Asparagus	Shredded winter squash
Broccoli	Cauliflower	Baked potato with skin
Spinach	Alfalfa sprouts	Snow or sugar snap peas
Onions	Pinto beans	Frozen peas, thawed
Tomatoes	Red cabbage	Red and green peppers
Kidney beans	Avocado	Garbanzo beans or chickpeas

- **Toppings** These can add extra crunch or zest to your salad, while being rich in nutrients.

Almonds	Sunflower seeds	Sesame seeds
Soy nuts	Ground flaxseed	Wheat germ
Raisins	Walnuts	Olives

- **Dressing** Avoid dressings containing large amounts of saturated fat and cholesterol. Watch out for hydrogenated fats on the ingredient list. Canola and olive oil are some of the best fats to have in a salad dressing. Most salad dressings are very high in fat, so you may wish to chose a low-fat variety. Or experiment with different vinegars, such as balsamic and rice vinegar.

Quick & Easy Dressing

1/3 cup red wine vinegar	1/8 tsp. garlic powder
1 cup extra-virgin olive oil	1/4 tsp. fresh ground pepper
2 tbsp. Dijon mustard	1/2 tsp. dried dill weed

Combine all ingredients in a covered container, such as a glass jar with a lid. Shake vigorously and pour to taste over your salad. Try not to drown your salad in dressing.

Using Sweeteners at Home

There are sweeteners that are better than the highly processed white sugars in many foods. **Sucanat, date sugar, stevia, rice bran sweetener, blackstrap molasses,** and **apple sauce** can all be used in baking in place of white sugar. By converting to these types of sweeteners you usually won't need as much and the body converts these into a useable fuel source more efficiently. This means less fat and a reduced effect for those with blood sugar problems. The easiest substitute is fruit juice. When cooking, 1/2 to 1 cup of apple juice or grape juice can be used. Whatever amount of juice you use, remember to reduce your milk substitute or water amount proportionally. A low calorie substitute for sugar is stevia. This is a sweet leaf from Brazil that can be used to sweeten drinks and baked goods. Finally, for sweetening baked foods, you can use 1/3 to 1/2 the amount normally used with cane sugar when using like sucanat, brown rice syrup, blackstrap molasses, fructose, or date sugar.

Eating Out and Traveling Tips

The streets of any city are lined with many restaurants for us to choose from. As many of us know, restaurant foods will never compare to what we can create at home! Many restaurants are not as educated nor creative with good nutrition and healthful eating.

Nevertheless, we all find it necessary or exciting to visit restaurants occasionally, whether it be for business or social reasons, and our health need not suffer. Surprising, many restaurants, whether Italian, Mexican, Chinese, American, or vegetarian, will include some healthful choices on their menus. With a little knowledge of the right questions and choices, we can make better choices while eating out. The key is to stick to the low-fat, high-carbohydrate, mainly plant-based plan. Following are types of places that will offer health-supporting choices, questions to ask before or while visiting these places, and alternatives to eating at restaurants. These guidelines will help you on a consistent road to better health.

Places to Choose

Vegetarian restaurants or snack bars in a health food store

- Menu may offer some nondairy, or nonfat dairy, no meat, low salt, and unrefined foods. These include grains, beans, peas, pasta, vegetable dishes, salads, soups, and combinations made with these healthful foods.
- Some offer full meals, others sandwiches such as Avocado-Tomato, Tempeh Burgers, and Pita with Vegetables and soups such as bean and vegetable.
- Not all foods in "natural" food restaurants are healthful. Avoid *too much* high-fat plant foods (nuts, seeds, peanut butter, avocado) as well as *too much* animal foods and refined foods.

Restaurants with salad bars and/or baked potatoes

- All fresh vegetables and fruits are healthful.
- Avoid prepared dishes at the salad bar (macaroni salad, oily mixtures, combinations with mayo, canned fruits, etc.). Stick to the fresh foods.
- Choose a balsamic vinaigrette dressing, although many restaurants' are high sugar, and chemicals. Another alternative is to use lemon and/or oil and vinegar dressing.
- Use fresh veggies (mushrooms, broccoli, chives, etc.) and salsa for baked potato toppings instead of high saturated fat foods such as cheese, sour cream, and butter.
- Some salad bars also offer pasta cooked in very little oil. Top this with a marinara sauce and fresh vegetables (mushrooms, broccoli, tomato, carrot, etc.).
- Take your own non-hydrogenated margarine for potatoes.

Specialty restaurants with no MSG (monosodium glutamate), low salt, no animal fat choices. (Many restaurants carry low-oil vegetarian entrees.)

- *Italian restaurant*—choose spinach or whole-grain noodles if possible with a marinara sauce (usually this sauce contains low or no oil, is low calorie, and is made fresh at the restaurant). Avoid or limit cheese or dairy sauces, as they are high in fat.
- *Mexican restaurant*—choose those Mexican places that do not cook beans in lard. Limit the cheese and sour cream because they add too much fat to your entree. Choose tostadas, burritos, or tacos made of tortillas, fresh vegetables, salsa, and beans.
- *Chinese, Thai, and Japanese*—choose low-oil, low-salt, no MSG entrees. Choose brown rice if available. These restaurants should be called first to inquire about the MSG and salt. Some will make entrees to order without oil.
- *American restaurants*—basic steak-and-potato restaurants will most likely offer salad bar and baked potato, but try asking for a special dish to order. Many elegant dining restaurants will offer vegetable-rice or pasta dinners cooked to your preference, so ask for no dairy or MSG. Also, many times double helpings of potatoes, vegetables, and grains such as brown rice, whole-grain bread, and cereal can be ordered when other ingredients (buttery sauces, sour cream, and cheese) are left out.

Restaurants for a good breakfast

- Ideally choose places with whole-grain pancakes, waffles, muffins, bagels, hot cereals, and bread.
- Choose whole-grain water bagels (not cooked in butter) from a bakery or bagel shop.
- Avoid high-fat breakfast foods such as eggs, bacon, butter, sausage, omelets, and greasy hash browns.

- Use fresh fruit in hot cereal (apple, raisin, banana, etc.), use fruit or syrup on pancakes and waffles, and use fruit or jelly or almond butter on bagels, toast, and muffins, and limit topping any of these breakfast foods with butter, margarine, cream cheese, or whole milk.
- Fruit juices are best consumed if diluted with water to decrease the simple sugar concentration. Fruit smoothies are a tasty nutritional way to consume fruit. You may substitute soy milk for the juice to decrease the sweetness.

Avoid fast-food and other restaurants that specialize in high-fat, low-fiber meals. These include McDonald's, Jack in the Box, hamburger and hot dog stands, etc. However, some greasy fast-food restaurants do offer salads and baked potatoes now if you find yourself there.

Alternatives to Restaurant Eating

- Pack a lunch, even to a business meeting or event.
- Fruits and vegetables may be purchased at local grocery store for an occasional quick lunch.
- Before going to a party or dinner that serves junk food, have a meal at home, thus avoiding temptation. This is good advice to parents for children also.
- If all else fails, missing one meal never hurt anyone.

Questions to Ask (On the phone or while ordering)

- What vegetarian or low-fat entrees are available? Is there oil or dairy in them? How much? (Depending upon where you stand on the continuum of oil, a teaspoon of oil may not be worth skipping the dish).
- Do you have brown rice? (Not colored white rice, but whole-grain rice). Is it cooked in water, oil, or butter?
- Is there oil or lard in the refried beans? If oil, is it canola?
- Is there oil, lard, or dairy in the sauce or soup?
- Is there MSG or salt, a concern if you have high blood pressure, in the dish (especially Chinese)?

Now you are ready to eat out healthfully wherever you may be. Good luck on your road to better health!

Suggested Cookbooks for Eating In!

Amazing Grains, Joanne Saltzman
The American Vegetarian Cookbooks, Marilyn Diamond
The Complete Vegetarian Cookbook, Karen Brooks
Cooking for Life, Cherie Calborn
Cooking with Natural Foods, Black Hills Health & Education Center
Country Life (magazine, kitchen recipes)
Diet For a Small Planet, Francis Moore Lappe
Fit for Life, Marilyn Diamond
Fit or Fat Recipe Book, Covert Bailey
Fit or Fat Target Diet, Covert Bailey
Friendly Foods, Brother Ron Pickarski
The High Road to Health, Linsey Wagner
Home Cooking, Linda McCartney
Kathy Cooks . . . Naturally, Kathy Hoshijo
May All Be Fed, John Robbins
The McDougall Plan, John A. McDougall
The McDougall Plan Recipes, Mary McDougall
Mousewood Cookbook, Mollie Katzen

The Natural Foods Sweet Tooth Cookbook, Eunice Farmilant
New York Times Natural Foods, Black Hills Health & Education Center
Nutrition Almanac, John D. Kirschmann
The Pritikin Diet, Nathan Pritikin
Sweet and Natural, Janet Warrington
Vegetarian Times (magazine—great recipes)
Fields of Greens, Annie Somerville
The Enchanted Broccoli Forest, Mollie Katzen
The Raw Gourmet, Nomi Shamon
Rolling Prairie Cookbook, Nancy O'Connor
Raw, the UnCook Book, Juliano
Completely Vegan, Debra Wasseman

Sometimes eating out can be more nutritious than eating at home, especially when it comes to finding a restaurant as conscientious as ***Native Foods*** of California. The following is one of their menus (Westwood version), permission granted to print by owner and Chef Tanya Petrovna.

WESTWOOD MENU

Earth Bowls

Chinese "save the" Chicken Salad (Soy) 7.95
Romaine, cabbage, grilled soy chicken, Jasmine rice, corn, green onions with a light sesame orange vinaigrette

Native Caesar Salad 6.95
Romaine, homemade garlic-rubbed croutons and our own Caesar dressing. Add blackened soy chicken or tempeh 1.50

Jamaican Jerk Salad 8.50
Jerked seitan atop Jasmine rice and romaine with flamed banana salsa.

Killer Weed Salad 9.50
Carrots, onions, sprouts, cucumbers and seaweed topped with roasted hemp nuts and tofu with Island dressing crisp salad greens.

Eat-It-Raw-Mama Salad 8.75
Chopped raw veggies tossed with salad greens, cabbage, sprouts, yellow beets, avocado garnish, manna bread, balsamic vinaigrette.

Rojo y Mojo 7.50
Warm black beans and salsa tossed with balsamic vinaigrette over salad greens with tortilla chip croutons. Add brown rice... 1.00

Iron Yam 8.95
Steamed yam halves on salad greens topped with steamed veggies and marinated tofu with balsamic vinaigrette.

Soy Amigo 7.50
Our version of a taco salad. Salad greens, cabbage, soy taco meat, salsa, tortilla chip croutons. Corn, cilantro, green onion garnish. Soy good with avocado... 1.25

Mini-Greens Salad 3.95
Romaine, yellow beets, sprouts, onions and carrots topped with sunflower seeds, croutons and balsamic vinaigrette. Excellent as a side salad.

Hot Bowls 9.75

Hollywood
Brown rice, steamed veggies and marinated tofu spears with our tangy peanut sauce. Oh Soooo L.A...

Gandhi
Jasmine and brown rice, steamed veggies and blackened tempeh topped with cranberries and our wild curry sauce. Promotes world peace.

Mad Cowboy
Barbeque sauce-marinated soy chicken skewers grilled vegetables, baked potato, topped with ranch dressing and green onions. A Texas favorite.

Ray's Macro
Macrobiotics in a bowl. Brown rice, quinoa, tempeh, steamed veggies, cucumber and sea veggies with sauerkraut garnish and sesame sauce.

Rasta Pasta Primavera
Rigatoni pasta, steamed veggies and jerked seitan cubes covered in marinara sauce topped with roasted garlic croutons and pesto garnish.

Soba Dan Dan
Japanese buckwheat noodles and steamed veggies topped with green onions, sesame seeds, tangy peanut sauce and blackened tempeh.

Rockin' Moroccan
Skewered soy-chicken nuggets marinated in our spicy ginger Moroccan marinade atop grilled veggies and quinoa garnished with currants and almonds.

Bongo Congo
Wild curry-marinated soy-chicken skewers over steamed veggies and Jasmine rice topped with curry sauce.

Native Pizza

Spike's BBQ 8.95
Barbequed soy chicken, caramelized onions, cilantro, Native Cheese and barbeque sauce on thick-crust pizza dough.

The Greek 9.95
Marinara, mushrooms, caramelized onions, pommodoro, Kalamata olive seitan, pesto and Native Cheese on thick crust pizza dough.

Soups

Daily Soups—inquire 3.50

Native Chili 4.75
Topped with Native Cheese and onions. Served with cornbread.

Handholds

Bali Surf Burger 6.25
What we're famous for! Tanya's sauteed and grilled tempeh, lettuce, tomato, red onion and mayo on a whole wheat bun.
Blackened... .50 Caramelized Onions ... .50 Mushrooms... .75 Native Cheese... 1.00 Guacamole... 1.25

Jerk Burger 6.95
Jamaican-Jerk-marinated seitan steak, lettuce, tomato, red onion and mayo on a whole wheat bun.

Reu"Bruin' Burger 7.95
Blackened tempeh, sauerkraut, Native Cheese, lettuce, tomato, red onion and Island dressing on a whole wheat bun.

Spicy Soy Chicken Burger 6.50
Blackened soy chicken breast, Island dressing, lettuce, tomato, red onion and mayo on a whole wheat bun.

BBQ Love Burger 6.95
Thin slices of seitan slathered with BBQ sauce, caramelized onions and sprouts on a whole wheat bun.

Malibu Veggie Burger 7.25
A Native original veggie burger made with soy, quinoa, oats, veggies and delicious seasonings. On a wheat bun with sprouts, tomato, Thousand Island. Makes waves!

Philly Peppersteak Sandwich 8.25
Our sliced and seared peppered seitan, sautéed mushrooms, caramelized onions, bell peppers and Native Cheese, a French roll.

Moby Dick Sandwich 6.95
Battered and flash fried tempeh, surfer sauce, lettuce, tomato and red onion on a whole wheat bun. A"dick"tive!

Poltz Burrito 7.50
Seared seitan, brown rice, black beans and banana salsa in a wheat tortilla with guacamole and salsa fresca garnish. Rocks hard!

Tijuana Tacos (2) 6.75
Soy taco meat, salsa fresca, Native Cheese, shredded romaine lettuce and guacamole on grilled corn tortillas.

Baja Surf Tacos (2) 6.95
Battered and flash fried tempeh, surfer sauce, salsa fresca, shredded cabbage and guacamole on grilled corn tortillas.

Palm Springs Wrap 7.25
A best seller from home... Tanya's tempeh salad, jasmine rice, shredded lettuce, carrots, tomato, sun sprouts and a balsamic drizzle in wheat flat-bread.

Texas Hound 5.95
A flamed-broiled veggie dog in a wheat bun covered with Native chili, Native Cheese and red onions.

GET (the) FRIED Chicken Burger 6.95
Soy of course, with lettuce, tomato, onion and mayo on a whole wheat bun.

Snacks

Indonesian Tempeh Chips 4.95
Battered and fried tempeh strips served with your choice of sweet soy, ranch or barbeque sauce. Extra sauces. 50.

Native Seasoned Fries 2.75
Fried in vegetable oil and lightly seasoned with a Native blend of spices.

Get 'Yo Greens 3.75
Steamed organic leafy greens with your choice of balsamic vinaigrette or sesame sauce. Get 'yo calcium, iron and magnesiYum!

Edamame 3.50
Steamed soy beans dusted with sea salt.

Native Nachos 6.95
Tortilla chips topped with black beans, soy taco meat, Native Cheese, salsa fresca, guacamole, corn and green onion garnish.

Chili Cheese Fries 5.75
Native seasoned fries covered in Native Chili, Native Cheese and chopped red onions.

Thai Sticks 4.95
Sautéed and grilled tempeh satay served with peanut sauce.

"Save the" Chicken Wings 4.95
Our soy chicken battered and fried with ranch to dip. Too hip.

Sweet Treats

Seasonal Fruit Cobbler 4.00
Fresh fruit with a granola-crumb topping.

Native Carrot Cake with Frosting 4.00
The rage!

Elephant Chocolate Cake 4.00
Served with cinnamon peanut butter icing.

Key Lime Parfait—Tang for your bang! 4.00

Hollywood Cheesecake 4.00
New York never had it this good.

Boogie Bar 3.00
Wheat flour, bananas, almonds, oats, coconut and chocolate chips. Native decadence.

Drinks

Native Iced Tea—Caffeine-free hibiscus tea sweetened 1.50 with apple juice.

Fountain Sodas 1.50

Guru Chai—Black tea, soy milk, unrefined sugar and spices. 2.75

Assorted Bottled Juices 3.50

*Dinner menus vary slightly

**Not every ingredient is listed. If you have a specific food aversion, please check with a Native. Native Cheese is made with rainforest cashews and sunflower seeds. Entire menu is nondairy, even mayo! All tempeh and seitan homemade by Native Foods! The Best!

chapter 15

Energy Metabolism—Converting Food to Energy

Chapter 3 explored the basics of digestion and absorption. Metabolism is the next step in the process from food to energy. Although there are varied caloric needs among athletes (from 2,000 Calories a day for some golfers to 15,000 Calories a day for some Race Across America bicyclists), energy can be stored or used, and every cell in every human body requires energy. As explained in chapter 1, energy can be measured by units of energy (usually a Calorie or kilocalorie). The energy content of food is measured by bomb calorimetry, and a Calorie is the heat required to raise 1 gram of water 1 degree Centigrade. The body absorbs 92%–100% of this energy. The rate of energy metabolism is measured either directly (which requires many hours of testing an individual in an isolated chamber) or indirectly by measuring the rate of energy expenditure through the O_2 and CO_2 exchange during exercise or at rest.

A Bomb Calorimeter for Measuring Food Energy

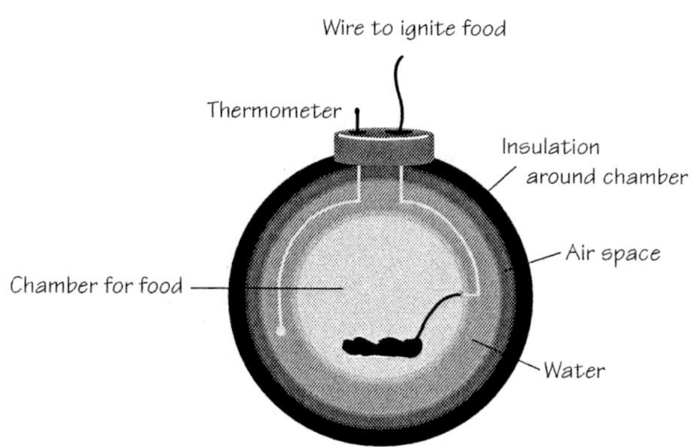

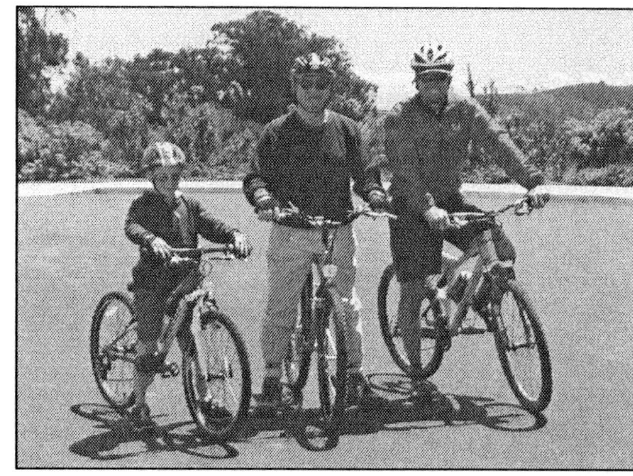

Different Ages Require Varying Caloric Needs

Human Metabolism and Energy Balance

Human metabolism is all the physical and chemical changes that occur in the body. The metabolic rate is how fast or at what rate the body uses its energy stores. The basal metabolic rate (BMR) is the metabolic rate at rest and is taken after 12 hours of fasting. The resting metabolic rate (RMR) is the same as the BMR, but not at rest or fasting (one may have had previous activity). The resting energy expenditure (REE) is the RMR plus environmental factors that could alter metabolism such as the cold. Another component of metabolism or energy expenditure is the thermic effect of food or TEF, which is usually about 10% of the total Calories consumed. Exercise and metabolism are a third component of energy expenditure called exercise metabolic rate (EMR) or thermic effect of exercise (TEE).

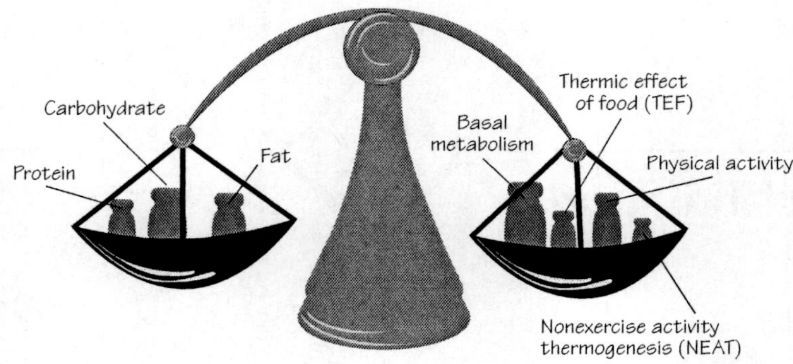

Adding the three components together equals your total energy expenditure for the day. Usually the BMR or REE (basic metabolism component) is the largest burning component unless you engage in long endurance exercise that brings the physical activity component up to a percentage greater than or equal to the basal metabolism.

Food contributes basically three sources of energy, which are carbohydrates, protein, and fat, that can be stored in the body or utilized for energy. Carbohydrates can be stored as glycogen and circulates as glucose. Proteins can be converted to glucose for energy as a last resort. Fat can be stored in an endless abundance as stored fat.

How Energy Is Stored and Used in the Body

The mitochondrion of the cell is the place of oxidation in the cells and the powerhouse of where most oxygen is consumed. Exercise increases the number and size of the mitochondria. **ATP (adenosine triphosphate)** is the energy current in all cells. Carbohydrates, fat, and protein convert to glucose, then pyruvate, then acetyl COA, then enter the **Krebs cycle** (named after Sir Hans Krebs and also called citric acid and TCA cycle) and with oxygen and ADP produce ATP and carbon dioxide. The anaerobic system yields 2 units of ATP per unit of glycogen and the aerobic energy system yields 36–38 units of ATP. All of this is only possible with the help of many vitamins and certain minerals.

Vitamins and Minerals Are Key Coenzymes in Metabolism

Muscle cells utilize the energy provided by fats, carbohydrates, and protein. Carbohydrates provide liver fuel and tissue fuel, continual glucose for the brain, and glucose concentration in the blood that must be maintained. Stores can only be maintained by continuous carbohydrate intake, not protein and fat. Glycogen cannot switch muscles, and those muscles specifically trained will store more gly-

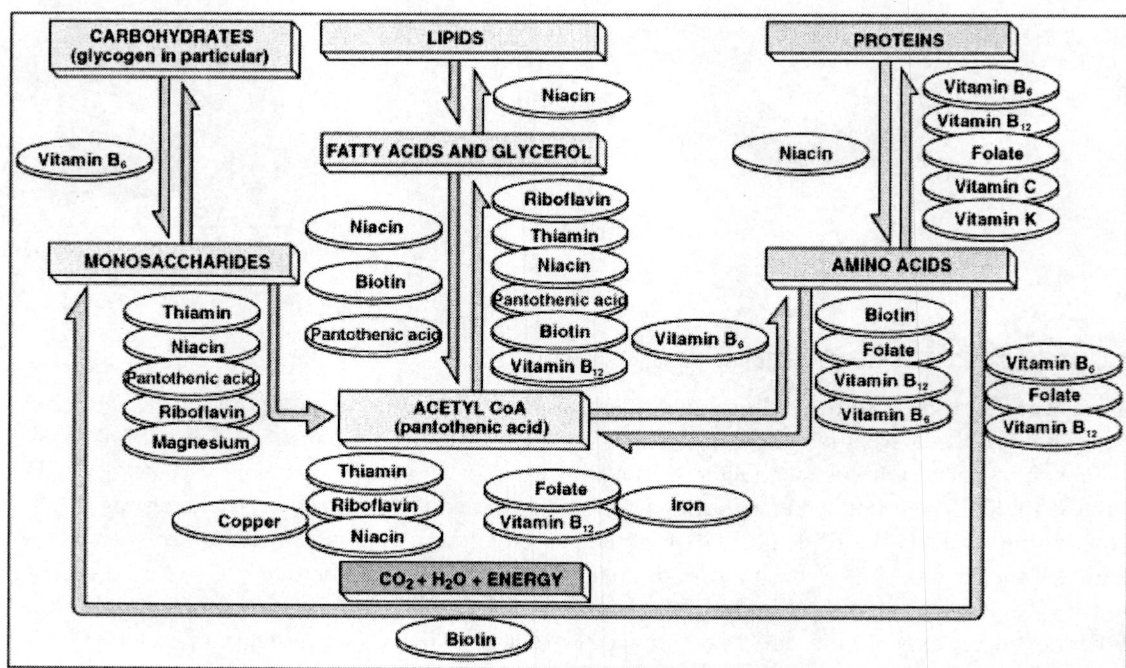

cogen. Protein does not store for muscle fuel, but is continually being synthesized and broken down into amino acids for cell functioning. Amino acids synthesize into protein for liver processes or structure, amino acids are released into the blood for the muscle tissues repair and growth, and they may be used for energy through the process of **gluconeogenesis** (making of new glucose), which is less efficient than carbohydrate energy use. When protein is used for energy, the nitrogen is eliminated (converted to ammonia and excreted with water through the blood and kidneys), then the remaining carbon skeleton is converted to glucose for tissues that need it. They may provide missing pieces if glycogen stores are becoming depleted, or the carbon skeleton may be converted to fatty acids and stored as triglycerides in the body's fatty storage areas of adipose tissue. Fats may be stored directly as triglycerides and when excess glucose or protein is not used by the body stores as fat, the process is called **lipogenesis** (the building of fat).

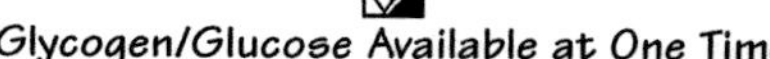

Glycogen/Glucose Available at One Time

50 kcal in the blood
250–300 kcal in the liver
1400–1500 kcal in the muscle

1700–1850 Total (trained athletes can double in muscle cells)

How Energy Transfers into Muscular Activity

Muscle fibers can be divided into three categories, depending on their color and preference of speed of twitching. **Type 1 (slow oxidative or slow twitch)** are usually used during endurance sports and are reddish in color representing the increased oxygen flow. **Type 11a (fast oxidative glycolytic)** are pinkish in color and are used during intermediate activities such as the 800 meter run. **Type 11b (fast glycolytic or fast twitch)** are white and are used in more anaerobic type activities and sprinting. Muscle fibers are used or recruited generally in the order of SO, then FOG, then FG. Muscle fiber contraction is believed to involve the proteins actin and myosin contracting in the myofibrils, then calcium ions releasing in the sarcoplasm of the cells with nerve impulses that stimulate muscle contraction. This is called the sliding filament theory.

In each cell, energy is used by the removal of a phosphate (ATP-ADP) every time the muscle contracts. At rest, ATP transfers from fat to muscle. When beginning exercise, ATP is generated from CP (creatine phosphate). At steady-state exercise (comfortable, but steady aerobic starting at about 5–15 min.), the cell's fuel comes from *carbohydrates* from the muscle and liver and *fats* from the muscle and FFA (free fatty acids) in the blood. The CP pool is resynthesized for later. A mixture of substrates (use of CP, carbohydrates, or fats) occurs at any one time, and there is no switching at depletion if you run out of one (muscles will not switch fuel to one that runs out and running out of glycogen will not lead to a total fat use mode). Fat is energy for most ATP resynthesis because it is so abundant in the body.

Fuel Use During Varied Exercise

Different percentages of each fuel are used during exercise, depending on several factors such as exercise intensity and exercise duration. Glycogen is always being used. At a low intensity during exercise, there is a mixture of fat, glucose, and glycogen. At submaximum intensity, there is mainly carbohydrates and lactic acid used. At a maximum intensity, creatine phosphate is used, and lactate will be formed at maximum after the 10–15 seconds of CP utilization. The most rapid and greatest glycogen depletion occurs during short-term exercise. After a steady-state has been reached, glycogen accounts for about 50%–60% of fuel needs, and the rest is fat. During a marathon, about there is about 50% fatty acid utilization.

Additional factors that affect which fuels are used and ultimately how energy converts to muscular activity are exercise type and one's training status. For team games (intermittent activity), more glycogen is spared than the same activity without recovery. Many metabolic changes take place when a person trains (exercises), such as a greater density of mitochondria (increase in oxidative enzymes), increased capillarization (increase blood supply to muscle), increased gluconeogenic capacities of muscle and liver, and increased cardiac output to working muscle. A trained individual uses more fat and increases performance by his or her ability to work at a higher rate with same previous fatigue level.

The preceding diet and prolonged exercise also affect how energy goes into muscular activity. Low carbohydrate stores will lead to an inability to support resynthesis of ATP. High carbohydrate store increase one's endurance capacity. Eating simple sugars before competition may cause one to use glycogen stores early in an event, and caffeine may cause a high proportion of fat burning over glycogen burning during competition (although it is also a diuretic). During prolonged endurance exercise there is a mixture of fat and carbohydrate burned for fuel. In the first 5–10 miles of a run, a mixture of carbohydrates and fat are burned for fuel (45%–50% glycogen). Fatigue will occur when energy cannot keep up with demand, usually from lack of glycogen storage. In summary, without adequate carbohydrate consumption, glycogen is depleted, fatigue occurs, and performance is greatly hindered. The next chapter gives specific recommendations of carbohydrates to delay fatigue and their role in competition.

Summary of Major Characteristics of Muscle Energy Systems

	ATP-CP	Lactic Acid	Oxygen (Carbohydrate)	Oxygen (Fat)
Main energy source	ATP, CP	Muscle glycogen	Muscle glycogen	Muscle fats
Exercise intensity	Highest	High	Lower	Lowest
Rate of ATP production	Highest	High	Lower	Lowest
Power production	Highest	High	Lower	Lowest
Capacity for total ATP production	Lowest	Low	High	Highest
Endurance capacity	Lowest	Low	High	Highest
Oxygen needed	No	No	Yes	Yes
Anaerobic/aerobic	Anaerobic	Anaerobic	Aerobic	Aerobic
Characteristic track event	100-meter dash	800-meter run	5- to 42-kilometer run	Ultramarathon
Time factor at maximal use	1 to 10 seconds	30 to 120 seconds	More than 5 minutes	Hours

Causes of Fatigue During Exercise

Fatigue is a very complex phenomenon. It is often classified as either psychological or physiological, but the two are usually related. The site of fatigue may be in the central nervous system (brain or spinal cord) or the peripheral, located in the muscle tissue or nerve-muscle junction itself. In sports nutrition, fatigue is defined as the inability to continue exercising at a desired level of intensity. The most important factor in the prevention of fatigue during exercise is training. Athletes must train the specific energy systems specific to their event, and because nutrition plays an important role in each of the energy systems, nutrition plays a key role in fatigue.

The intensity and duration of exercise determines this nutrition–fatigue relationship. The following levels of activities are listed with their most probable causes of fatigue.

Type of activity	Cause of fatigue	
Mild aerobic exercise (long distances)	Low blood sugar Dehydration Excessive mineral loss	(Body fat stores are sufficient for fat portion but glucose needed to burn the fat)
Moderate to heavy aerobic (especially over 90 min.)	Muscle glycogen depleted Low blood sugar Dehydration	
Very high intensity exercise	Excess lactic acid in muscle Low muscle glycogen stores	
Extremely high intensity (lasting only 5–10 sec.)	Depletion of phosphocreatine	

In addition to the preceding causes of fatigue, a deficiency of almost any nutrient may be the cause of fatigue. A poor diet can hasten the onset of fatigue. Proper nutrition is essential not only to access the energy of carbohydrates and fat, but also for the metabolism of protein, vitamins, minerals, and water. See the carbohydrate and carb-loading sections for detailed recommendations. See chapter 4, "Carbohydrates," and chapter 16, "Nutrition for Training and Competition," for detailed recommendations.

chapter 16

Healthful Nutrition for Training and Competition

The Energy Demands and Essential Nutrients for the Athlete

Athletes are concerned with whether they are getting the needed nutrients to support training and performance. The 45 essential nutrients can be obtained from the diet or if necessary (as in the case of illness, injury, or eating disorders) from supplements. Although protein, carbohydrate, and many vitamin and mineral needs are increased for athletes, these can be easily attainable through the increase in Calories that athletes consume to support energy balance. The main difference between athletes and nonathletes is the amount of Calories consumed. The daily energy needs of the individual athlete are largely determined by body weight and the energy demands of their specific sport. Low-energy-demanding sports such as golf, baseball, and bowling may increase daily caloric requirements 5%–15% about nonactive levels. In contrast, endurance sports, like running, bicycling, and swimming, may increase daily caloric requirements by 50%–100%. An athlete should be aware of the relative energy demands of her/his exercise and training time (see "Personal Assessments," chapter 19). The next step is designing a diet that is 65%–75% carbohydrates, 10% protein, and 20% fat. Lack of the proper amount of Calories or an imbalance in the percentage of Calories can cause general fatigue, apathy, and declining body weight or slowed growth—all of which add up to less-than-optimal performance.

The DRIs have been established to give people the amounts that they need of each nutrient as a daily average. It is recommended that you average at least 3–5 days to calculate your daily nutrient intakes because food and liquid intakes vary from day to day. DRIs have not been specifically established for athletes because their needs vary so greatly, depending on the sport, sex, body weight, and individual goals. However, consuming 150% of most of the key micronutrients (vitamins and minerals) should cover extra needs. Macronutrient needs can be estimated more closely; therefore, this chapter will emphasize carbohydrate, protein, and fat needs for athletes.

General Guidelines and Food Guides for Active People

Number of exchanges for each diet

Daily Calories	~3000	~4000
Starch	19	26
Vegetable	7	9
Fruit	6	9
Nonfat, 1%, or soy milk	3	3
Lean protein	3	4
Fat	9	13

The general dietary guidelines and food guides explained in detail in chapter 2 can be applied to the athlete's diet as well. Athletes and active people could use any pyramid to serve as a basic guide, but they would most likely benefit most from the non-USDA pyramids that focus on more plant-based high-complex carbohydrate foods such as the Healthful House of Food and Fitness and the Mediterranean Diet Pyramid. If using the USDA pyramid, athletes would need to add food servings to each category in a proportional manner (i.e., add starches and veggies first before the protein and "dairy" categories and keep those still to a minimum to keep protein and fat from becoming excessive). Athletes may also use the exchange list system to make day-to-day meal planning easier than adding each of your energy nutrients daily. The exchange lists are designed to ensure that you get a specific amount of Calories and energy nutrients (fat, carbohydrates, and protein), whereas you are able to choose which foods you want to eat as long as you adhere to the serving amounts and the number of servings (exchanges) from each category. Remember that the system does not ensure that you will make the most nutritious choices for vitamins and minerals and phytochemicals (i.e., it does not distinguish between organic whole barley and a white roll). The table in chapter 2 shows the exchange categories, the energy nutrients of each category, and sample food plans to meet these needs. For athlete examples, a female athlete may need 3000 Calories a day and a male athlete may need 4000 a day. The number of exchanges has been taken from the table in chapter 2, and a sample diet plan is given in the table (varied serving amounts and sizes for each individual). The exchange list numbers are designed for the athlete to obtain a 62%–65% carbohydrate/13%–17% protein/20% fat breakdown.

A Healthful Day of Eating for an Athlete

Use the Exchange Lists for Portions and Adjust for Caloric Choice (Note the Nutrient Dense and Photochemical-Rich Choices)

Breakfast:	Whole-grain hot cereal w/blueberries, papaya, and soy milk Fresh grapefruit juice
Lunch:	Tempeh burger on whole wheat bun w/lettuce, tomato, pickle, nayonaise mustard/mayo Raw carrots w/hummus dip
Dinner:	Whole wheat penne pasta with white bean/marinara sauce Mixed green salad w/cherry tomatoes, yellow bell pepper, avocado, purple onion (balsamic dressing) Steamed asparagus w/roasted garlic Fresh multi-grain bread
Snacks:	Fruit smoothie w/banana, flax seed, frozen strawberries, crushed ice, and rice milk Organic popcorn

Carbohydrates for Training and Competition

Carbohydrates are the most readily available and digestible form of energy for the athlete, making it the most crucial nutrient for them. Energy production is the prime function of carbohydrates. You read in chapter 4 all about the types of carbohydrates and in chapter 15 about the metabolism of carbohydrates. Dietary carbohydrates, sugars and starches, are converted into glucose in the body for fuel to maintain the blood sugar level. The athlete draws on stored carbohydrate (glycogen) for energy use during exercise. Glycogen can sustain work to about 2 hours, and once it is depleted, the body can only work at about 50% of maximal capacity (this type of fatigue is called "bonking" or "hitting the wall"). Workouts will train the muscles to store more glycogen. Unlike glycogen, blood glucose levels can only be sustained for about 30 minutes. Ingesting 30–60 grams of carbohydrate per hour of strenuous endurance exercise can delay fatigue.

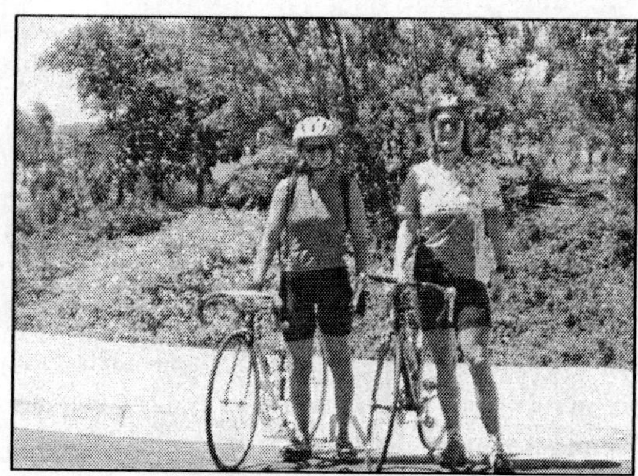

Training Is More Fun with Friends

Daily Carbohydrate Requirements for Varied Training Regimens

Daily CHO requirements gms/lb weight	Training Regimen	Goals	Sample Athlete: 125 pounds	Sample Athlete: 165 pounds
2.5–3.0 gms/lb	Moderate duration Moderate intensity Under 1 hour Low intensity, several hours	Daily muscle glycogen recovery	280–375 grams	370–495 grams
3.0–4.5 gms/lb	Prolonged Moderate–high intensity Daily > 90 minutes	Daily glycogen muscle recovery Refueling during exercise Load muscle for exercise	375–562 grams	495–742 grams
4.5–5.5 gms/lb	Very prolonged Moderate–high intensity Daily > 5–6 hours	Daily glycogen muscle recovery Refueling during exercise Meet high energy needs	563–690 grams	742–907 grams

Daily and Postexercise Carbohydrates for Selected Body Weights

Body Weight in Pounds	Postexercise Carbohydrate Requirements .5 to .7 grams/lb/day	Daily Carbohydrate Requirements 2.25 to 5.5 grams/lb/day
100	50–70 grams	225–550 grams
110	55–77 grams	248–605 grams
120	60–84 grams	270–660 grams
130	65–91 grams	292–715 grams
140	70–98 grams	315–770 grams
150	75–105 grams	338–825 grams
160	80–112 grams	360–880 grams
170	85–119 grams	380–935 grams
180	90–126 grams	405–990 grams
190	95–133 grams	428–1045 grams
200	100–140 grams	450–1100 grams

Precompetition Carbohydrates

The preevent dinner, eaten about 15 hours prior to competition, should consist of foods that you are used to and foods that are primarily carbohydrate (preferably the fresh, unrefined complex type such as vegetables, whole grains, and fruits). A general formula for long strenuous competition is to consume 8–10 grams of carbohydrate for every kilogram you weigh for the preceding 3–5 days before the event, especially the day before. (Remember to find your kilograms by taking your pounds and dividing by 2.2). For example, if you weigh 135 pounds, then 135/2.2 equals 61 kilograms of body weight. If you multiply 61 times 8, then you need a minimal of 488 grams of carbohydrates the day before competition. Because there are 4 Calories in a gram of carbohydrate, you would need almost 2000 Calories the day before competition to be from carbohydrate. This is why fat and protein are kept at a minimal level on these days so that Calories will not be excessive in the process of adding carbohydrates. To get 488 grams of carbohydrates, you can eat several small meals throughout the day of whole grains, whole-grain products, fruits, and veggies (with small amount of lean proteins, if any, because the whole-grain foods alone would add up to enough protein in the quantity eaten).

Carbo-Loading: The Healthful Way

"Carbo-loading" is a common term among athletes that has many definitions. To some, it simply means to increase carbohydrates before a big event. There is a traditional method and a more modern or healthful method of carbohydrate-loading for important endurance races.

The traditional method of carbo-loading, first practiced by the Scandinavians, included a low-carbohydrate diet for several days, then a high-carbohydrate diet during the rest days. This was effective in glycogen supercompensation (going beyond normal preexercise glycogen levels), but may result in ketosis (a condition in which fats are incompletely broken down into ketones and may disturb the body's normal acid-base balance and lead to other health problems). Other negative effects of the traditional method are low energy for training and dehydration because of the lack of water stored with glycogen. The studies of athletes utilizing the traditional method have only tested up to 19 miles of running. One other problem is that most athletes could not increase the carbohydrates 40% over their normal diet to benefit from the very low carb days.

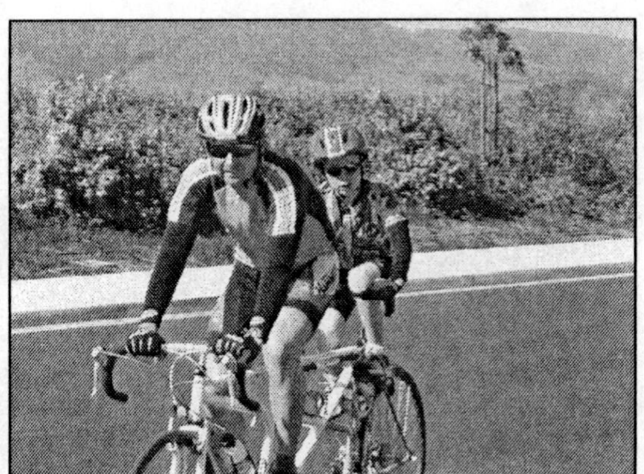

Double Your Fun on a Tandem

The modern method of carbo-loading is to consume a normal carbohydrate diet (of about 300–500 grams of carbs a day) for a few days, then a high-carb diet during the 3–5 rest days preceding the event. This method is just as effective in glycogen supercompensation, without the negative effects. Studies suggest that the most effective amount of grams is 500–600 during this high-carb period. This amounts to 2000–2400 Calories of carbohydrates (4 Calories per gram), therefore leaving little room for fat and protein Calories beyond what naturally is available in healthful complex carbohydrate foods. These foods should come mainly from the bottom three portions of the pyramid—whole grains, vegetables, and fruits.

The "modern" method of carbo-loading, in practical terms, is actually the recommended high-carb diet (70%–75% of total Calories from complex carbohydrate) with an increase in the same types of foods before a race. It is not nearly as beneficial for an athlete to eat steak every night, then pasta the night before a race. Just as important as the prerace meal is complex carbohydrates immediately following the event (the power hour for glycogen repletion) and high-complex carbs in the following 24 hours. Studies show recovery time is greatly enhanced.

Research tailors the gram amounts to each athlete, depending on body weight. It also sheds some light on the timing and amount of carbs for long events (i.e., marathon). Studies also show that trained females may not need as much as trained males because of their more efficient use of fatty acid utilization for energy. Therefore, females may use the lower end of the range.

Carbs Before the Race

If you are susceptible to reactive hypoglycemia (low blood sugar caused by eating simple carbs), then avoid eating any simple sugars 15–60 minutes before an event. This especially applies to the consumption of sports drinks.

At 5–10 minutes before a task that will be over 2 hours, a carb feeding has been shown to help delay the onset of fatigue and improve performance if the exercise is above 60%–75% of max. A more concentrated carb solution may be taken then.

At 4 hours before a long race, the ingestion of 4–5 grams per kg of body weight has been shown to be effective. Because each gram of carb equals 4 Calories, this would amount to about 240–300 gms of carbs, or 1200 carb Calories for a 132-lb. person for a prerace meal. (Keep in mind that there is some fat and protein even in most high-carb foods, so this may mean a 1400-calorie breakfast). This is more than most people are used to, but very effective in loading the liver and muscles with glycogen to last all the way to mile 26 in a marathon.

At 1 hour prior to a race, 1–2 grams per kg of body weight is effective.

Carbs During a Race

With normal liver and muscle glycogen stores, carbohydrate feedings are unnecessary for bouts 60–90 minutes or less.

Sometime between 90–120 minutes, carbohydrate is needed to allow fat burning to continue, to maintain blood glucose levels, to reduce the psychological perception of effort, and to prevent early slowing of pace.

As the muscle glycogen falls, the need for the amount of ingested carb for energy increases. Even a single feeding late in a race may help replenish blood glucose levels, increase carbohydrate oxidation, and delay fatigue!

If you are running at 65%–85% of your VO_2 maximum, then 1 gram per minute of carb energy can be derived from your blood glucose. This amounts to about 6–8 oz. of a 6% carb solution every 15–20 minutes to maintain glucose levels. Ultramarathoners may ingest a 10%–20% solution of carb concentration.

Carbs After

After the event, 8–10 gms per kilogram per day is important for glycogen replenishment (preferable in a combo protein/carb food such as beans, rice, etc.).

A Recommended Carbohydrate-Loading Program

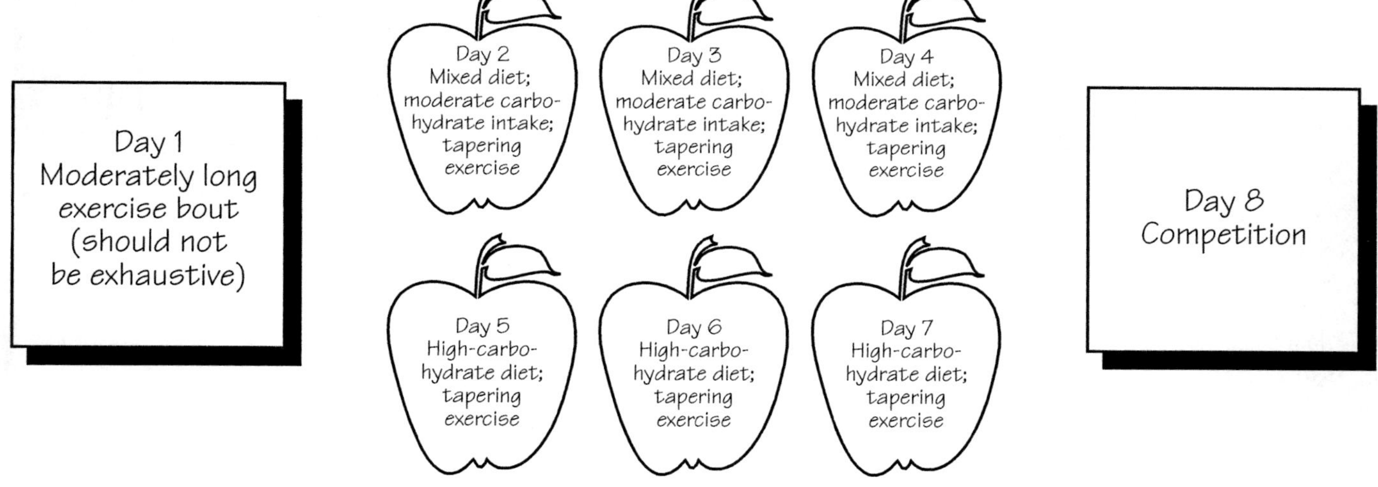

Note: The moderate carbohydrate intake should approximate 300–500 grams of carbohydrate per day; the high carbohydrate intake should approximate 500–700 grams per day.

Sample Race Day Food and Liquid Plan for a Selected Athlete in a Half Ironman (2k swim/56 mile bike/13.1-mile run)

Sample Athlete

- 155 pounds
- 70 kilograms
- Recommend: 4–5 g/kg wt.
- 280–350 grams of carbohydrates in prerace meal (1120–1400 kcal)

Race Breakfast

2 bowls shredded wheat w/rice milk (76 grams)
1 banana (28 grams)
5–6 strawberries (15 grams)
1 cup juice (23 grams)
Bagel w/jam (76 grams)
1 cup yogurt (24 grams)

Total carbohydrate grams = 242 grams (968 Calories of CHO)
+ Gel hour and 15 minutes before race (40 grams)

Total carbohydrate grams = 282 grams (1128 Calories of CHO)

During Race

.6 g/kg wt. per hour = 42 grams per hour for 70-kg athlete

1000 Calories

42 grams of carbs per hour

250 grams of carbs for race

10 Gels plus some sports drinks

Drink 2–3 cups of fluid per hour, which is 1.5 water bottles.

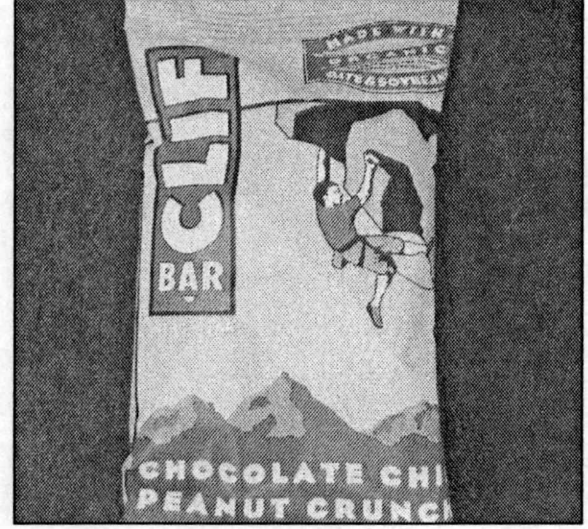

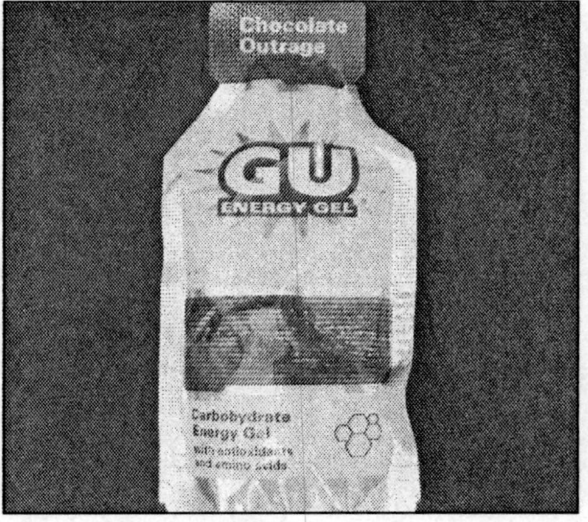

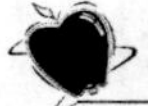

When to Eat During Race

Race Time	Number of Gel
:45 (transition area or on bike)	1
1:15 (bike)	2
1:45 (bike)	3
2:15 (bike)	4
2:45 (bike)	5
3:15 (bike—before transition)	6
3:45 (run)	7
4:15 (run)	8
4:45 (run)	9
5:15 (run)	10
Any more as needed for more time past 5:45.	Make sure to drink water with all Gels!

Proteins for Competition

Although athletes need large amounts of carbohydrates to work, they also need protein to build and maintain muscle. Protein is found throughout the body in every cell and is necessary to produce enzymes that participate in the body processes and to make hemoglobin, the oxygen carrier. Proteins are also important for an athlete's fluid balance and producing antibodies to fight off infection.

Careful food choices, such as following the Healthful House of Food and Fitness, will lead to a diet free of high-fat protein foods and excessive protein. By eating meats and dairy, the fat percentage of the diet is often increased. By eating nonfat animal products, the daily protein intake is greatly increased and often excessive. As mentioned in chapter 6, too much protein may lead to osteoporosis and kidney and liver problems.

Because it takes a long time and much biochemical work for protein to become muscle and provide any appreciable energy for the body to use, stocking up on protein just before competition will not do you much good and may have an adverse effect. A common belief among athletes and coaches is that protein needs are greatly increased with training, especially with strength-developing exercise. However, hard training does not increase the percentage of protein or specific amino acids. The protein gram requirements will increase some for athletes trying to increase the size and strength of their muscles, but the recommended guideline of .8 grams per kilogram of body weight still meet most athletes' needs. Some bodybuilders and endurance athletes will benefit from consuming 1–1.5 grams per kilogram of body weight, as shown in chapter 6. Although protein only provides 2%–5% of energy needs during rest and low to moderate exercise, it provides 10%–15% of energy needs during endurance exercise. Hard exercise increases protein needs by activating specific enzymes in the muscle that degrade the myofibrillar protein, and protein loss through sweat and urine occurs because of decreases absorption in kidney tubules during heavy exercise.

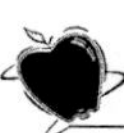

Recommended Protein Intakes in Grams per Kilogram Body Weight for Sedentary and Physically Active Individuals

	Grams of protein/kg body weight
Sedentary	0.8
Strength-trained, maintenance	1.2–1.4
Strength-trained, gain muscle mass	1.6–1.8
Endurance-trained	1.2–1.4
Weight-restricted	1.4–1.8

The values presented represent a synthesis of those recommended by leading researchers involved in protein metabolism and exercise.

To calculate body weight in kilograms, simply multiply your weight in pounds by 0.454. Then, multiply your weight in kilograms by the appropriate value in the grams per kilogram body weight column to determine the range of grams of protein intake per day. Teenagers should increase this amount by 10%.

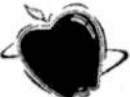

Total Daily Protein Needs of a 70-Kilogram (154-Pound) Athlete

Authority	**Recommendation (g/kg/day)**	**Protein/Day (g)**
Food and Nutrition Board (RDA)	0.8	56
ADA/CDA	1.0–1.5	70–105
Lemon, P.W.R. (endurance athletes)	1.2–1.4	84–98
Lemon, P.W.R. (strength-speed athletes)	1.2–1.7	84–119

Sources: Position of the American Dietetic Association and the Canadian Dietetic Association: Nutrition for physical fitness and athletic performance for adults, *Journal of the American Dietetic Association* 93 (1993): 691–695; P.W.R. Lemon. Effect of exercise on protein requirements, in C. Williams and J. T. Devlin, eds., *Foods, Nutrition and Sports Performance: An International Scientific Consensus* (London: E & FN Spon, 1992), pp. 65–86.

Fat for Competition

Fat serves as a less-efficient energy source, a supplier of essential fatty acids, a carrier for fat-soluble vitamins, and an insulator of the body's organs. If fat is ingested prior to competition, fatigue and poor performance is likely. It takes a minimal of 3–5 hours to digest a fatty meal, therefore avoid any concentrated fats prior to competition. Examples of fatty foods are the unhealthful fats such as butter, hot dogs, French fries, fried foods, bacon, sausage, hamburgers, whole milk, and dairy ice cream. Also avoid healthful fats in the 3 hours prior to competition, such as nut butters, oils, and avocados.

Vitamins and Minerals for Athletes

Vitamins and minerals are involved in many body metabolic processes such as growth, repair, bone structure, fluid balance, blood building, and the release of energy from food and the body's store (see tables in chapter 8). Vitamins and minerals are considered micronutrients because although each has an essential role in the body, a very small amount is necessary to accomplish these roles. Vitamins and minerals are measured in micrograms and milligrams instead of the grams that the energy nutrients are measured.

Dietary deficiencies of vitamins and minerals have been shown to impair performance, yet there is little evidence that they will improve performance when taken ergogenically in excess. Supplements are not required if you are eating a nutritious diet. Specifically, wholesome carbohydrates such as vegetables, whole-grain cereals, and whole-grain breads contain the B vitamins. Most fresh fruits have vitamin C. Red and green peppers, potatoes with skins, lima beans, brussels sprouts, and broccoli contain both B and C vitamins. Bok choy, chard, broccoli, and kale are excellent suppliers of iron and calcium. Dark leafy green vegetables, pumpkin, squash, carrots, whole grains, beans, cabbage, cantaloupe, and watermelon contain optimal amounts of vitamin A, K, and E. The sunshine helps our bodies to produce vitamin D.

Common Nutrition Questions of Athletes

1	Q	What should I eat the night before a competition or event?
	A	*It depends on whether the event is longer than 2 or 2.5 hours. If it is longer, then the carbo-loading worksheet should be used for accurate amounts of carbs and calories. If it is shorter, then typical high-carb dinners are sufficient. Drink lots of water.*
	Example	*Whole-grain pasta with marinara sauce (small amounts of concentrated protein such as lean meats, tempeh, or tofu) • Whole-grain rolls or bread (spectrum canola spread is one of the most healthful butterlike spreads) • Steamed veggies • Salad (low-fat or nonfat dressing)*
	Example	*Whole-grain tortilla (Trader Joe's good) • Brown rice • Black beans or low-fat refried beans • Dairy cheese or soy cheese (small to moderate amounts) • Any veggies • Avocado or guacamole*
2	Q	What should I eat the morning of competition or a workout?
	A	*Once again, it depends on the time and the length of the event, but breakfast is always a must! A general guideline is to eat between 300–500 Calories of high-carb foods if you have 1.5–2 hours before the event/workout. Eat 500–800 Calories if you have 3 hours to digest the food. Events or workouts that are longer than 2 hours may need a 1000–1500 Calorie breakfast, depending on your weight and fitness level.*
	Example (~500 Calories)	*Whole-grain cold cereal (TJ Shredded Spoonfuls, Puffins, Shredded Wheat, etc.)—1 serving • Nonfat milk or Rice Dream Brown Rice Milk (TJ has) • Banana • 3/4 glass O.J.*
	Example (~500 Calories)	*Whole-grain bagel (with unsweetened jam or apple butter) • Oatmeal—1 serving • 3/4 glass O.J.*
	More High-Carb Examples	*TJ Pastry Poppers • Whole-grain toast • Whole-grain muffins/waffles/pancakes • Fresh fruit (papaya, mango, strawberries) • Fresh fruit smoothie • Yogurt (dairy or soy)*
3	Q	What should I snack on in-between events/matches/games or shortly before a workout in the middle of the day?
	A	*Carbohydrates are still the key. Some people can eat simple carbs better than other people can right before a workout or competition. Experiment to see what works best for you. Eat easily digested foods and avoid too much fat or protein because they will sit in your stomach. Cow's milk should also be avoided right before competition. Drink water.*
	Examples	*Bananas/oranges/apples • Dried figs (diced at TJ)/date pieces • Crackers/pretzels/WW bagels/healthful muffins • Clif Bars (others similar—avoid hype of high-fat/high-protein) • "Gels" like "GU" for most easily digested form • Sports drinks if diluted 6% and tolerable (glucose polymer/fructose combo best)—not recommended for young children. Water is best.*
4	Q	What should I eat after competition or a hard workout?
	A	*Eating a high-complex carb/moderate protein meal within an hour is ideal. At least eat a bagel or some other grain food to hold you over until a meal can be eaten. Muscle glycogen stores will be replaced more fully if this guideline is followed.*

Competition Guidelines Table

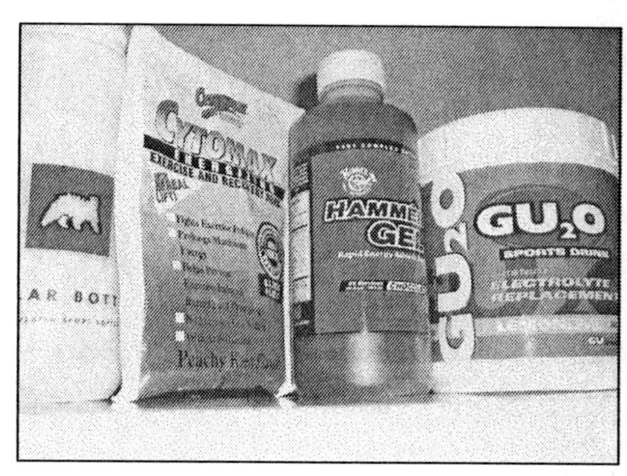

Competition guidelines have been given such as carbo-loading, protein needs, fluid needs, ultramarathon needs, and meal plans and food ideas. During endurance competition, protein and fat during the race do not need to be consumed in large quantities. Your breakfast will meet your protein and fat needs until dinner after the race. During ultramarathon events (cycling 200 miles, swimming the English Channel, or running 100 miles), a food replacement drink may be used to obtain all of the six classes of nutrients. GUs and sports drinks will get you through a race up to 6–10 hours, and then food replacement shakes may be beneficial for satiety, satisfaction, and other nutrient losses.

Competition Guidelines for Foods and Fluids

	Months Before Race	Day(s) Before Race	Hours Before Race	During Race	After Race
Foods/Carbohydrates	Check with race officials which foods and sports drinks will be offered at race.	Follow carb guidelines (8–10 grams of carbs per kg of body weight each day 3–5 days before race). Generally 500–700 grams carb/daily for most people.	Follow carb guidelines for weight (generally 200–300 gms carbs in premeal). Choose foods you are used to. Drink calories if digesting food is difficult before race.	Consume 30–60 grams of carb per hour of the race or .6 grams of carb per kilogram per hour. (A 165-pound male divided by 2.2 equals 75 kilograms times .6 equals 45 grams of carb per hr. of race or 225 grams for 5 hours.)	Consume a protein/carb ratio of 1:4 (20 grams of protein to 80 grams of carbs) after exercise.
Hydration	Practice drinking during exercise.	Hydrate with water frequently (remember, every extra gram of glycogen stored will store 3 grams of water, so you may gain a pound of water daily during glycogen-loading (will benefit you in heat).	Drink about 2 cups of water 2 hours before the race.	Sports drinks should contain a 6% carb concentration to avoid pulling water away from the cells back into the lumen of the small intestine and dehydrating you.	Drink water to rehydrate.
Gels/Tapering/More Specifics	Experiment with different energy bars, gels (Hammergel, Powergel, GU) and sports drinks while training.	Taper your training as you glycogen load with an easy week before the race.	Choose foods low in fat and protein for quicker stomach emptying.	Drink 6–8 oz. every 15 minutes. Calculate carb calories from sports drink and gels into total carb grams for event (drink 16–24 ounces per hour, which is 2–3 cups; if 12 oz. consisted of a sports drink at 6% solution then the total carbs from the sports drink would be 22.5 grams, leaving 22.5 grams from a gel or food).	Pack foods for postrace such as bagels with almond butter or cheese or a yogurt or baked tofu on whole-grain crackers.

The Competitive Edge

Athletes are bombarded by supplement companies, advertisements, and sometimes coaching recommendations to try a particular product. Nutritional quackery, as introduced in chapter 1, is rampant in the sports nutrition field because top athletes that are similar in genetics and equipment are looking for the competitive edge, and supplement manufacturers want to profit from this attitude. Athletes are often looking for an ergogenic aid—meaning a substance that will produce more work and a better performance. There are pharmaceutical (i.e., steroids), psychological (i.e., visualizations), biomechanical (aerobars for cycling), physiological (blood doping), and nutritional (excess chromium or iron) substances that athletes may try for an ergogenic effect. Athletes should be forewarned that often these aids act as placebos in which they may seem to work because the athlete mentally gets a boost from them. It is also possible that the athlete was deficient in the substance, and it worked because the body was no longer deficient (such as with iron deficiency). Also keep in mind that many of these substances can cause dangerous side effects. Buyer beware!

The following table gives common ergogenic substances used in sport with their effects and risks.

Ergogenic (*energy-giving or work-producing*) Substances in Sport

Ergogenic Aid	***Claim***	***Effectiveness***	***Risk***
Anabolic steroids (male sex hormone)	Used to promote muscle growth	Generally effective for muscle gain during exercise	Many, including heart disease, kidney and liver problems, and death
Androstendione (male hormone)	Similar to the above, but still legal in some sports	May be effective for muscle growth; elevates testosterone and estrogen in males and females	The same effects are possible as with anabolic steroids
Arginine and ornithine (Nonessential amino acids)	Claimed to enhance secretion of human growth hormone, the breakdown of fat, and the development of muscle	No increase in growth or lean mass	High levels of amino acids may interfere with the absorption of others
Bee pollen (a product of bee saliva, plant nectar and pollen)	Claimed to help recovery from training	No evidence of a recovery benefit	Some individuals have allergic reactions
Bicarbonate (baking soda/alkaline salt)	Claimed to help buffer lactic acid produced during exercise	Increase in blood pH that may enhance performance and strength in anaerobic activities	"Soda loading" may cause bloating, diarrhea, and a higher blood pH
Caffeine (stimulant)	May produce alertness and reaction time and increase the release of fatty acids from adipose tissue, which will spare glycogen and enhance performance	Some reports claim increased endurance	Dehydration, jitters, headaches, trembling, fast heart rate, digestive discomfort, delirium, and death
Carnitine (a nitrogen-containing compound formed in the body from lysine and methionine)	Helps transport fatty acids across the mitochondrial membrane. Claims to also burn fat and spare glycogen	Studies show no increase in fatty acid utilization or improvement in exercise performance	L-carnitine has little risk, but D, L and D-carnitine can be toxic
Chaparral (antioxidant)	Claimed to delay aging and cleanse the bloodstream	Unproven claims	Shown to cause acute toxic hepatitis
Chromium picolinate (an essential trace mineral)	Claimed to increase lean body mass, decrease body fat, and delay fatigue	Positively affects insulin action on energy nutrient metabolism, but will not affect this process unless there is a deficiency	Possible link with muscle degeneration
Coenzyme Q_{10} (a lipid found in cells)	Claimed to improve exercise performance	Studies shown it is effective for heart disease patients, but not healthy athletes	Unknown
Colostrum (first mammalian milk)	Claimed to improve exercise performance	It is "liquid gold" for babies to have their mother's colostrum, but no effectiveness for adults	Unknown
Creatine (nitrogen-containing compound that combines with phosphate to burn a high-energy compound stored in muscle)	Claimed to enhance energy and stimulate muscle growth	Studies are contradicting	Edema and nausea

(continued)

Ergogenic (*energy-giving or work-producing*) Substances in Sport (*continued*)

Ergogenic Aid	Claim	Effectiveness	Risk
DHEA Dehydroepiandrosterone (hormone made in the adrenal gland that serves a precursor to the male hormone testosterone)	Claimed to burn fat, build muscle, and slow aging	Ineffective according to studies	May have similar effects as steroids over a long period of time
DNA and RNA (deoxyribonucleic acid and ribonucleic acid—the genetic materials of cells)	Claimed to help protein synthesis by taking extra	The body produces enough to do protein synthesis; extra does not improve this process	Unknown
Ginseng (a stimulant herb)	Claimed to spare glycogen, increase fatty acid oxidation, and reduce fatigue	No human research to support these claims	Nervousness, confusion, depression, insomnia, and high blood pressure
Glycine (nonessential amino acid)	Claimed to help anaerobic activities	No proof	May cause an imbalance of other amino acids
Growth hormone (hormone naturally produced by brain's pituitary gland to regulate growth)	Promoted to cause an increase in lean body mass	Sometimes works in older people and those needing the hormone	Causes carpal tunnel syndrome and other tissue/nerve problems
Guarana (reddish berry found in Brazil that contains 7 times more caffeine than coffee)	Claimed to enhance speed, endurance, and memory	No studies completed	Stresses the heart and cause panic attacks
Inosine (an organic compound)	Claimed to activate cells, produce energy, and facilitate exercise	Studies show a reduction in endurance of runners	Unknown
Ma huang (herbal preparation—contains ephedrine)	Promises weight loss and increased energy	May act as a stimulant	A cardiac stimulant with many serious adverse effects such as headache, insomnia, nausea, vomiting, heart attack, stroke, and sudden death
Medium-chained triglycerides	Claimed to provide energy to bodybuilders without promoting fat deposition and reduce muscle protein breakdown during prolonged exercise	Energy that must be metabolized before stored as body fat. No human studies support claim	None known
Octacosanol (an alcohol extracted from wheat germ)	Claimed to enhance athletic performance	No proof	Unknown
Phosphate salt	Claimed to enhance cells potential to deliver oxygen to muscle cells	Demonstrated to increase diphosphoglycerate in the red blood cells to do this	May cause calcium losses from bones
Plant sterols (lipid extracts of plants)	Claimed to enhance hormonal activity	No proof	Unknown
Pyruvate (3-carbon compound derived from glucose, certain amino acids, and glycerol)	Claimed to burn fat and enhance endurance	No proof of any needed beyond body's production	Intestinal gas and diarrhea
Royal jelly (produced by worker bees and fed to the queen bee)	Claimed to enhance athletic performance	Unproven claims	Possibly allergies
Superoxide dismutase (SOD-enzyme that protects cells from oxidation)	Claimed to help recovery	When taken orally, body digests and inactivates this protein so it is useless	Unknown
Vanadium (vanadyl sulfate)	Claimed to produce more rapid and intense muscle pumping for bodybuilders	No evidence to support a benefit for bodybuilders	Reduces insulin production

chapter 17

Fluids and Hydration for Fitness and Sport

Fluid Needs and Regulation of Body Temperature

The body is about 55%–60% water—two-thirds of which is inside the cells. A very delicate balance exists between the input (drinks and foods) and output (elimination of urine and feces and sweating) of water. Water is an essential nutrient that is critical for the proper functioning of all bodily cells and maintaining a normal body temperature of 98–100 degrees. The impact of water on workouts and sports performance is even more pronounced.

The average person needs about a quart of water for every 1000 Calories eaten. Therefore, a person eating a 2000-Calorie diet would need about 2 quarts (8 cups) of water daily. When fruits and veggies consumption are increased, then water consumption through food is increased, possibly requiring less of a need through liquids. Also when carbohydrates are stored as glycogen 3 grams of water will be stored per unit of glycogen (which can be helpful in hyperhydrating for an event). Once again, this has led people to think you will gain weight on a carbohydrate diet, but the weight gained from increasing carbs and not increasing calories is water.

The Electrolytes

Electrolytes such as sodium, potassium, chloride, calcium, magnesium, and sulfate will conduct an electrical current in a solution. They are important to maintaining proper functioning in the cells. Sodium, chloride, and potassium are the main electrolytes that are lost through sweating, although most of sweat is water alone. Only with excessive sweating for a prolonged period of time would elec-

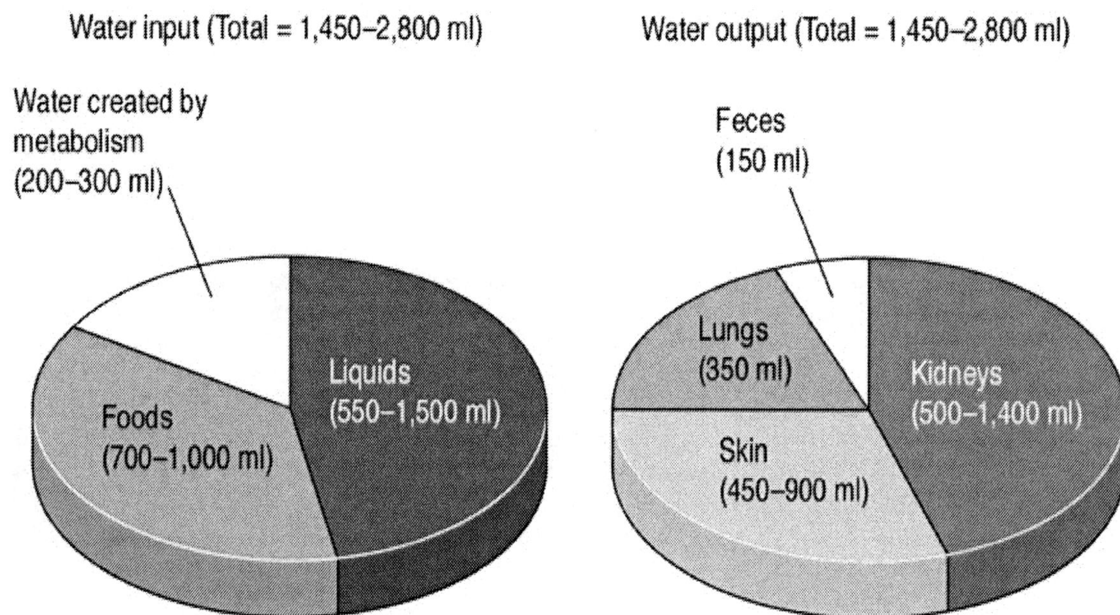

trolytes be lost to the point of needing supplementation. The daily requirement for these electrolytes and their food sources, functions, and deficiency symptoms are as follows.

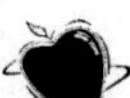

Electrolyte and Daily Requirement	Food Sources	Functions	Deficiency Symptoms
Sodium 500 mg	Plenty in whole foods (generally excessive in packaged foods, soy sauce, and added salt)	Fluid balance, nerve impulse conduction, muscle contraction acid-base balance, primary + ion outside of the cell	Hyponatremia, muscle cramps, nausea, loss of appetite, dizziness, seizures, shock, coma
Chloride 750 mg	Same as above	Primary – ion outside of cell, nerve impulse conduction, HCL formation in stomach	Rare—may be caused by excessive vomiting and loss of HCL, convulsions
Potassium 2000 mg	Potato, carrots, oranges, bananas, cantaloupe, mango	Same functions as sodium, but intracellular, glucose transport into cell	Hypokalemia, loss of appetite, muscle cramps, apathy, irregular heartbeat

Fluid Losses and Their Effect on Performance

If a person does not get enough water, then performance will be affected. Performance has been shown to decline at as little as a 2% of body weight water loss. At a 3% water loss, performance has been shown to decrease 10%. Sometimes athletes lose 8%–10% of their body weight. Symptoms may include dizziness, labored breathing, mental confusion, and spastic muscles at this loss. One should drink two cups of water for every pound of water lost (using the scale). Thirst is a poor indicator of water needs, so active people should drink water before, during, and after workouts and competition before becoming thirsty. The following chart gives symptoms that may occur with increased fluid loss.

Adverse Effects of Dehydration

% Body Weight Loss	Symptoms
.5	Thirst
2.0	Stronger thirst, vague discomfort, loss of appetite
3.0	Increasing hemoconcentration, dry mouth, reduction in urine
4.0	Increased effort for exercise, flushed skin, impatience, apathy
5.0	Difficulty in concentrating
6.0	Impairment in exercise temperature regulation, increased HR
8.0	Dizziness, labored breathing in exercise, mental confusion
10.0	Spastic muscles, inability to balance with eyes closed, general incapacity, delirium and wakefulness, swollen tongue
11.0	Circulatory insufficiency, marked hemoconcentration and decreased blood volume, failing renal function

Source: J. E. Greenleaf, W. J. Fink. Fluid intake and Athletic Performance IN *Nutrition and Athletic Performance* (W. Haskell, ed.). Bull Publishing Company, Palo Alto, CA, 1982.

Heat Exhaustion

- A depletion of blood volume from fluid loss by the body
- Body heat is lost primarily through evaporation of sweat
- Fluid loss through sweat is about 3–8 C per hour
- Humidity interferes with sweat production
- Decreases endurance, strength, performance
- Profuse sweating, headache, dizziness, nausea, weakness, visual disturbances

Sports Drinks

Although water is the largest constituent in sweat, sometimes it is necessary to replenish the sodium and potassium that is lost in excessive sweating in a hot environment. This is often achieved through the ingestion of sports drinks (also known as fluid-electrolyte drinks or glucose polymer solutions). Sports drinks may be beneficial for some athletes and active people. Water is the best drink for up to about 90 minutes of exercise. After 90 minutes (which can vary, depending on your last meal) blood sugar levels will fall, and performance will likely decrease from the fatigue that occurs with low blood sugar levels. A sports drink can raise blood sugar levels so that your body will continue to utilize glycogen (stored carbs) and utilize stored body fat for fuel. These energy sources cannot be effectively accessed with a low blood sugar level. Therefore, drinking something that will raise your blood sugar level delays fatigue.

However, not all sports drinks are created equal, and not everyone can handle them. Diabetics may not do well with them because of the high amount of simple sugars. Some athletes cannot ingest a sports drink before competition because it tends to cause a hypoglycemic type reaction, which leads to early release of glycogen and early fatigue. However, some athletes do well by ingesting a sports drink before an event, so you need to experiment before using them in competition. Most drinks are basically sugar, water, and sodium that you could make on your own. Some drinks use sucrose (a table sugar), and some use glucose polymers and fructose combined, which tends to work better. Fructose alone may cause gastrointestinal distress. The concentration of carbs in the sports drink is very important. If it is too concentrated, then osmosis will cause water to be pulled from the cells back into the lumen of the intestine, where the number of water molecules or concentration of the water is the lowest (basically dehydrating the cells). A 6% concentration seems to hydrate most effectively, which is about 15 grams of carb per cup of fluid. Juice has double this amount, so juice would need to be diluted by half with water. Sodas are the same as juice. Some sports drinks need to be diluted as well. Sodium, potassium, and chloride are the three electrolytes that may be lost in excessive sweating in a hot environment. Calcium and magnesium are also electrolytes. Small amounts of sodium help the sugar get absorbed more rapidly by helping with gastric emptying (from the stomach to the small intestine), and if athletes are exercising excessively in the heat, then they may be losing sodium. However, most people's diets contain 3–5 times the amount of sodium that they need. Potassium is more likely to be deficient in a diet that lacks fruits and veggies, but because sweat is mostly water, it is not usually needed in a drink. For ultraendurance events, all of these would likely be needed.

The main purpose of sports drinks are to delay fatigue by keeping blood sugar levels sustained so you can keep burning stored glycogen and stored fat for energy during exercise.

Heat Cramp
- Occurs in the skeletal muscle
- A complication of heat exhaustion
- Painful muscle contractions for 1–3 minutes at a time
- Ensure athletes have adequate salt and fluid intake
- Exercise moderately at first in the heat

Heat Stroke
- Internal body temperature reaches 105°F
- Symptoms: nausea, confusion, irritability, poor coordination, seizures, and coma
- Athletes should replace fluids and monitor weight change (fluid loss)
- Avoid exercising under hot, humid conditions

Comparing Fluid Replacement and Sports Drinks (per 8 oz. serving)

		Carbohydrate		Electrolytes (mg)	
Product	**Type**	**Grams**	**%**	**Na**	**K**
Red Bull	Sucrose (S), Glucose (G)	26	10	—	—
All Sport	High fructose corn syrup (HFCS)	19	8	55	55
Cytomax	Corn starch, Fructose (F)	13	5	53	100
1st Ade	HFCS, G, S, F	16	7	55	25
Gatorade	S, G, F	14	6	50	45
Hydra Fuel	GP, G, F	16	7	25	50
PowerAde	HFCS, GP	19	8	55	30
Quickick	HFCS	16	7	100	23
10-K	S, F	15	6	55	30
Orange Juice	F, S, G	25	10	6	436
Coca-Cola	HFCS, S	27	11	6	0
GU_2O	Maltodextrin, F	13	5	120	20

Sound Guidelines for Fluid Replacement and Keeping Cool

- Keep fluids accessible and cool (40–50 degrees).
- Hydrate well for air travel.
- Wear suitable clothing for hot or cold weather.
- Acclimatize to an area before competition there if hot.
- Avoid salt tablets—they may be harmful to the stomach and intestines, causing diarrhea.
- You should have four full bladders a day.

- In ultraendurance events, use CamelBaks, water sprayers, wet diaper hats, and white clothing to help regulate the body temperature in the heat.
- Avoid caffeine and alcohol that dehydrate.
- Avoid soda and straight fruit juice during competition.
- Use a 6% carbohydrate solution (15 grams of carb per cup of fluid).
- Drink 2 cups of water for every pound of body weight lost.
- Hydrate with water 20–40 minutes before exercise.
- Hydrate during exercise 3–6 oz. every 10–15 minutes.
- Hydrate after exercise; bring water because events do not always provide water.
- Larger volumes of water are absorbed more rapidly.
- Cool fluids leave the stomach more rapidly to be absorbed by the small intestine.
- Working above 75% of your maximum heart rate makes absorption more difficult.
- Drink before you are thirsty.
- Beware that some people react to sports drinks negatively, even at a proper concentration, experiencing nausea, stomach discomfort, dehydration, a blood sugar drop, and an increase in early glycogen release.
- Hyperhydrate before an event by drinking water frequently the day before the event.
- A combination of glucose polymers and fructose in a 5%–6% solution is generally most effective, but use water for up to 90 minutes of exercise.
- Choose purified water over tap water whenever possible.

chapter 18

Nutrition for Muscle Weight Gain

Nutrition Guidelines

When asked "Who wants to gain weight?" most people would not raise their hands. But if asked "Who wants to gain muscle?" many more hands are raised. Hardly anyone wants to gain fat, so most people have the same goals—lose fat, gain muscle. For some athletes such as in bodybuilding and strength-related sports, the goal of muscle gain is even more pronounced. The nutrition recommendations for weight gain is to gain 1 pound of lean body mass per week by increasing Calories, but keeping with the athletic recommendations of 20% fat, 10%–15% protein, and 65%–70% carbohydrate (mostly complex). Because there are 2300–3500 Calories in a pound of muscle, then theoretically athletes could gain a pound a week by increasing their Calories by 500 extra Calories per day. Strength athletes can use the same food guides and food exchange lists as other athletes.

The increased protein needed to achieve this muscle gain is about 14 grams extra per day because a pound of muscle is 454 grams, of which only 22% is tissue, or about 100 grams. Therefore, 100 grams of protein divided by 7 days is 14 extra grams of protein a day. Some male athletes attempting to gain muscle have needed as much as 1.5–1.75 grams of protein per kilogram of body weight, although most need only 1.0–1.2 grams of protein per kilogram of body weight. Either way, calories from protein can easily be met without supplementation or extra protein shakes if the athlete is eating the proper amount of Calories (see the Personal Assessment Worksheet for your personal needs).

For example, even a 200-pound male who weighs 91 kilograms would need a maximum of 159 grams of protein using the 1.75 grams per kilogram upper limit. The total Calories of protein would equal 636 (multiply by 4 Calories per gram), which would be 15% of 4242 Calories or 10% of 6360 Calories, thereby keeping the athlete in the 10%–15% protein range if he is eating this proper amount of Calories for his activity.

Exercise Guidelines

In order that the athlete does not put the extra 500 Calories to storing fat, resistance training must be included in the program to stimulate muscle growth. Resistance training should include preferably weight-training exercises that include large muscle groups. In order to work out at the strength end of the strength-endurance continuum, a low number of repetitions and high weight must be used for more muscle growth or hypertrophy. The type of equipment used can be either machines or free weights. The number of times you train each muscle group per week depends on the amount of exercise you plan to do for each body part and the amount of days you have to work out. The minimal is to work each body part (chest/back/shoulders/arms/legs) completely at least once a week, but ideally twice a week. Remember that muscle groups overlap, so if you are working chest and shoulders one day and back and biceps the next, then the bursa sac in the shoulder may become strained after repeated days of this routine. Completely resting the upper body every other day is not a bad idea. Crunches and vertical knee raises can be done daily for the abdominal area as long as no pain submerges from the hip flexor area from incorrect form.

Contraindications to weight training are high blood pressure and hernias. Aerobic exercise should not be eliminated in a strength program. Cardiovascular fitness is still the best health-related fitness component for heart health.

Rest Guidelines

In addition to nutrition and exercise, rest of the muscles and adequate sleep are equally important for muscle growth. Between sets it takes 2–3 minutes to restore most of the ATP and PC in the cells, and muscle protein synthesis can occur for up to 24 hours after a single bout of heavy exercise. It is important not to work the same muscle group two days in a row (the 48-hour rule) to allow the muscle growth to occur. Theories of muscle growth are increased water volume, increased muscle cells and myofibril size, increase in myofibril number, increased thickening of connective tissue around each muscle fiber and bundle, increased cell enzymatic and energy storage of ATP and glycogen, and increased number of muscle fibers themselves (which is less likely). Resistance training also increases bone mineral content, which decreases osteoporosis, which is more likely to occur in a sedentary person.

Caloric Intake for 150- to 160-Pound Male to Gain 1 Pound per Week

Caloric intake to maintain current weight	***2500 Calories (from Assessment Worksheet)***
Resistance Training Workouts ◆ 200 Calories per session ◆ 5 sessions per week	1000 Calories per week/7 = **143 Calories**
Aerobic Exercise ◆ 300 Calories per session ◆ 4 sessions per week	1200 Calories per week/7 = **170 Calories**
Muscle Tissue Synthesis ◆ 3500 Calories per pound	3500 Calories per week/7 = **500 Calories**
Total Caloric Needs	**3313 Calories**

chapter 19

Personal Assessments for a Fit Life

Ten personal assessments are designed to help you calculate your nutritional needs and increase your food choice awareness. You will need to enter 3 days of your food and liquid intake into the diet analysis software program and print out the average of your 3 days before completing these assignments and the overall dietary assessment in chapter 20.

The following assessments are included in this chapter.

1. **Food Guides—Which Is Right for You?**
2. **Carb Craziness**
3. **Lipid Love**
4. **Protein Panic**
5. **Micronutrient Madness (and Color Your Diet!)**
6. **EEE (Estimated Energy Expenditure)**
7. **Got FITT Program**
8. **When in Doubt, Throw It Out!**
9. **Food Label Savvy**
10. **Carbo-Loading Calcs**

After completing these assessments, you are ready for the final chapter, "A Personalized Evaluation and Plan"!

Name ____________________ Date __________

Food Guides—Which Is Right for You?

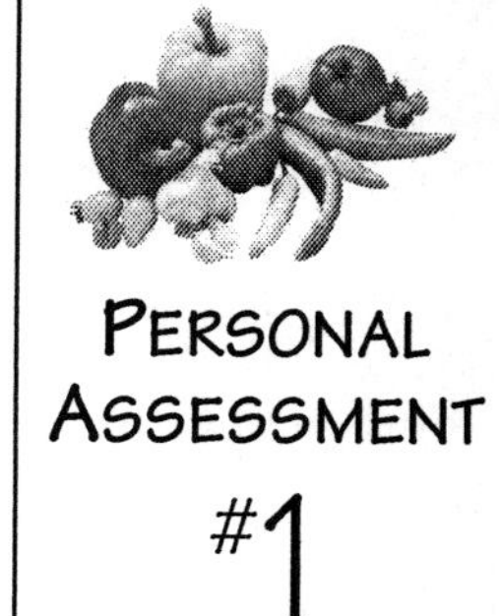

PERSONAL ASSESSMENT #1

Important—MyPyramid Tracking Sheet must be attached for any credit.

Look at the Food Guides in Chapter 2 and answer the following questions:

1. How much do *you* need from each category of the MyPyramid? (Attach MyPyramid.gov printout of recommended needs AND write below)

   Grains ______ Veggies ______ Fruits ______ "Dairy" ______ Protein ______

2. List the **foods** you ate today and **which category** they belong in on the **MyPyramid.gov Tracking Sheet** and attach to this paper.

3. Are you meeting all of your **recommendations**? Explain.

4. Explain the **quality** of your food choices in each section of the MyPyramid.

5. What do you **like** about the MyPyramid?

6. What **changes** would you make to the MyPyramid to make it more healthful?

7. How do the **other food guides compare** to the MyPyramid?

8. Which food guide would you say fits **your lifestyle and personal choices** best?

9. Using any **food guide**, explain a favorite **food** you would choose from each category.

   Grains ____________ Veggies ____________ Fruits ____________

   "Dairy"or Soy ____________ Protein ____________ Fats ____________

10. Could you eat as healthfully as **Healthful House of Food** recommends (i.e., all whole grains, every color category of fruit and veggie per day, etc.)?

Name ______________________________ Date ______________

Carb Craziness

(Go for those carbs! Don't avoid them!)

PERSONAL ASSESSMENT #2

Look at your diet analysis printouts

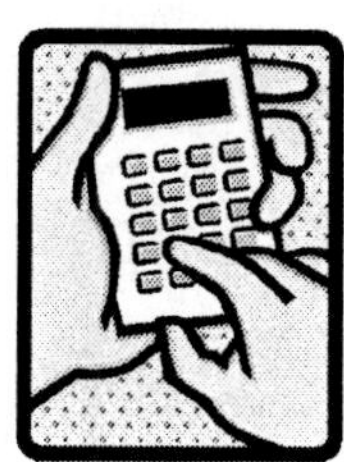

Record:

Total Calories ________

Carb grams ________

Fiber grams ________

Sugar grams ________

Fill in all the following blanks to calculate the total grams and percentage of carbohydrates.

Carbohydrate calculations:

Carbs: ________ g × 4 kcal/g = ________ Carb kcal

Carb kcal/Total kcal = ________ % carbs

Is this a minimum of 55%–65% of total kcal? ________

What percent of your carbs are simple? ________

Looking at the types of carbs you ate:

Is your fiber at least 25–40 grams per day? ________

Are your carbs mainly simple or complex? ________

Are your carbs mainly refined or unrefined? ________

Are your grains whole grain? ________

Is your diet plentiful in fruits and veggies? ________

How do you feel your carbohydrates can be improved?

____

Name ______________________________ Date ______________

Lipid Love

Love those good fats—but don't overdo it!

PERSONAL ASSESSMENT #3

Look at your diet analysis printouts

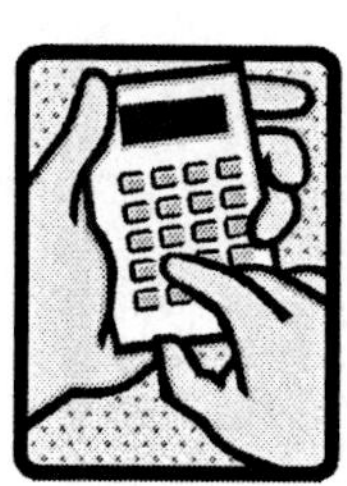

Record:

Total Calories ________

Fat grams ________

Saturated fat grams ________

Cholesterol milligrams ________

Fill in all the following blanks to calculate the percentages of fat and saturated fat.

Fat Calorie calculations:

Sat fat: ________ g × 9 kcal/g = ________ Sat fat kcal

Fat: ________ g × 9 kcal/g = ________ Total fat kcal

Fat percentage calculations:

% kcal from fat = ________/________ = ________
(Fat kcal/Total kcal)

% kcal from sat fat = ________/________ = ________
(Sat fat kcal/Total kcal)

Is your *cholesterol* under 300 mg? ________ (Zero is fine)

Is your *total fat* under 30% of total kcal? ________ (Preferably 20%)

Is your *sat fat* less than 7% of total kcal? ________ (Not essential)

Are there trans fats in your diet? ________

How do you feel your lipids can be improved? (Increase mono?)

____

Name ______________________________ Date ______________

Protein Panic

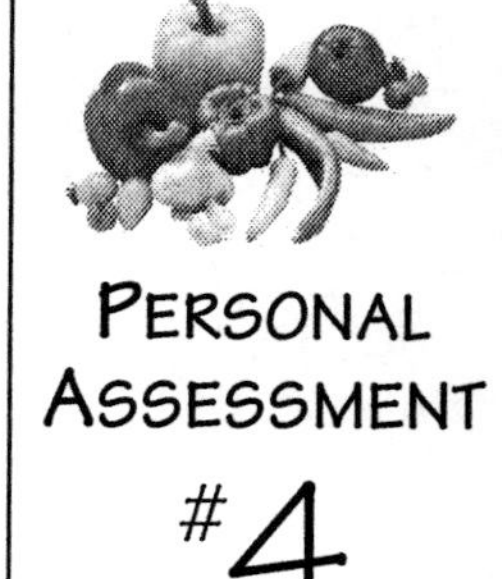

There is a panic to get more—most people get too much!

Look at your diet analysis printouts

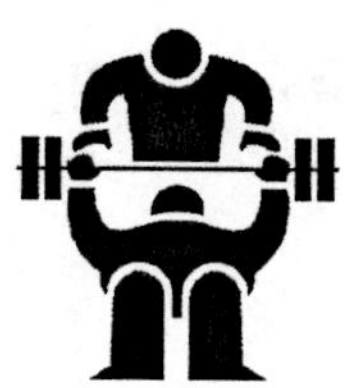

Record:

Total Calories ______

Protein grams ______

Fill in all the following blanks to calculate the total grams and percentage of protein.

Protein calculations (amount you ate):

________ Protein g × 4 kcal/g = ________ Protein kcal

(Protein kcal/Total kcal) = ________% kcal from protein

Is your protein 10%–15% of Calories? ________

(Percentages only a good tool if Calories are accurate for weight)

Protein calculated needs:

Record your body weight in kilograms (Pounds/2.2) ______

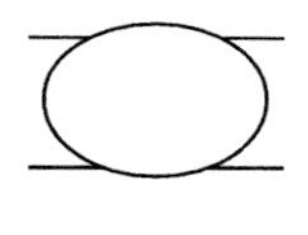

Multiply your weight by .8 for protein need ______

(DRI is .8 grams of protein per kilogram of body weight)

(Use 1.2 if you are a bodybuilder or endurance athlete)

How does the amount of protein you ate in the top box differ from your calculated needs in this box (see ovals)?

____

Name ______________________________ Date ______________

Micronutrient Madness

and color your diet!

PERSONAL ASSESSMENT #5

Look at your diet analysis printouts.

These are the **vitamins** listed on the diet printout:

A C D E K B_1 B_2 Niacin B_6 Folate B_{12}

Answer one of the following statements:

1. List the vitamins you are deficient in (less than 100% of the RDA). For *each* deficient vitamin, suggest foods that will improve the intake of that vitamin. Make sure suggestions are consistent w/macronutrient goals!)
2. If you were not deficient in *any* vitamins, give specific examples of why your diet is able to meet the RDA recommendations.

____

____

____

____

These are the **minerals** listed on the printout:

Calcium Iron Magnesium Phosphorus Potassium Zinc

Answer one of the following statements:

1. List the minerals you are deficient in (less than 100% RDA). For *each* deficient mineral, suggest specific foods that will improve your intake of that mineral. Make sure suggestions are consistent with macronutrient goals!
2. If you are not deficient in *any* minerals, give specific examples of why your diet is able to meet the RDA recommendations.

____

____

____

____

Phytochemicals

Look at the color in your diet. List the foods that you ate in your 3 days from each color of the dietary color wheel that are rich in phytochemicals that prevent disease. Write "None" if you do not have a fruit or vegetable in a particular category.

Red ______________________________

Red (Blue)-Purple ______________________________

Orange ______________________________

Orange-Yellow ______________________________

Yellow-Green ______________________________

Green ______________________________

White Green ______________________________

Name ______________________________ Date ______________

EEE (Estimating Energy Expenditure)

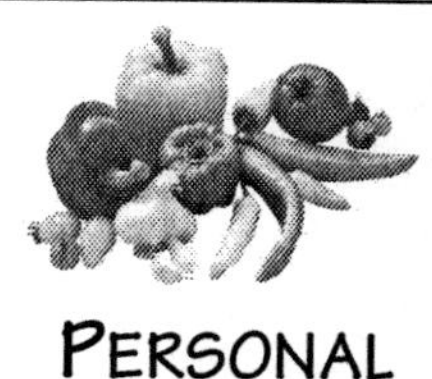

PERSONAL ASSESSMENT #6

Record the following:

Your weight in pounds ________

Your weight in kilograms (divide pounds by 2.2) ________

Hours spent asleep ________

Hours spent awake ________

Average Calories used per pound per hour (see following chart)—ACPH ________

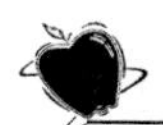

General Type of Activity	*Average Calories Used per Pound per Hour (ACPH)*
Sedentary (sitting most of day)	.23
Very Light Exercise (minimal movement)	.27
Light Exercise (2–4 hours/week)	.36
Moderate Exercise (4–7 hours/week)	.50
Severe Exercise (7–14 hours per week)	.77
Very Severe Exercise (> 14 hours per week)	1.00

Using the data from the top chart, calculate the following.

1. Basal Metabolism

a. Basal metabolism (24 hrs) = **1 × kg of weight × 24 hours**:

1 × ______ × 24 = ______

b. Saving in sleep = **0.1 × kg of weight × hours spent asleep**:

0.1 × ______ × ______ = ______

c. Subtract (b) from (a) to get basal metabolism Calories:

(a) – (b) = ______

Comment
Will equal ~ 10 x your body weight in pounds or 1000–2000 kcal

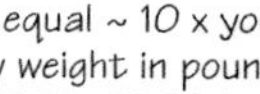

2. Adding Activity Calories

a. Calories for activity = **"ACPH" × weight in pounds × hours spent awake**:

______ × ______ × ______ = ______

b. Add basal metabolism Calories (1c) to activity Calories (2a):

______ + ______ = ______

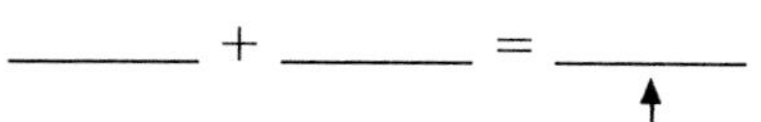

Comment
This will be more than basal metabolism!

3. Adding food tax (thermic effect of food) of 10%:

(2b) answer × .10 = ______

Estimated total Calories needed per day (2b + 3) for 3 components = ____________

Does this seem accurate for you? ______________________________

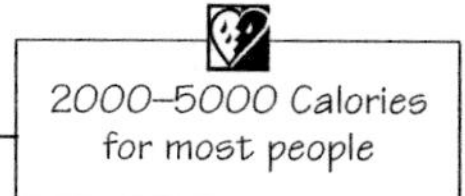

2000–5000 Calories for most people

Name ______________________________ Date ______________

Got FITT Program

PERSONAL ASSESSMENT #7

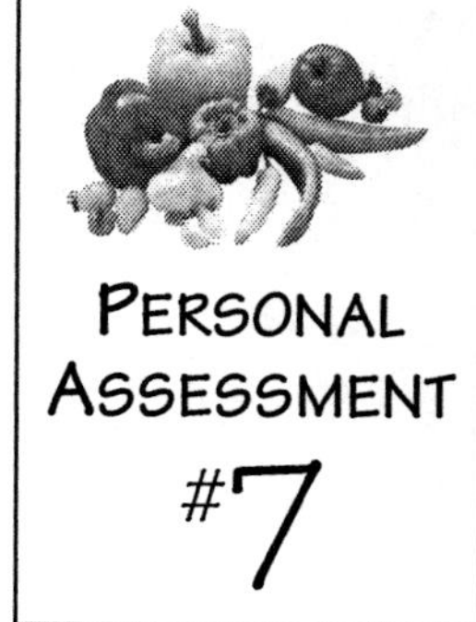

Plan your fitness program using the following chart.

The minimal ***Frequency*** per week is given: Fill in your ***Intensity*** level planned, the specific ***Type*** of activity, and amount of ***Time*** in each box to complete the chart utilizing the ***FITT*** Formula for exercise and all of the health-related aspects of fitness.

	Sunday	**Monday**	**Tuesday**	**Wed.**	**Thurs.**	**Friday**	**Sat.**
Flexibility (minimum 2x) ◆ Stretch ◆ Yoga							
Muscular Endurance (minimum 2x) ◆ Push-ups ◆ Crunches							
Strength (minimum 2x) ◆ Weights ◆ Machines							
Cardiovascular Endurance (minimum 3x) ◆ Run ◆ Swim ◆ Bike ◆ Fast walk							
Leisure Fitness (minimum 1x) ◆ Golf ◆ Kid play ◆ Rec sport							

Are you doing this schedule? Are you exercising 1 hour per day? ______________

Name ____________________ Date ____________

When in Doubt, Throw It Out!

Test Your Food Safety Knowledge

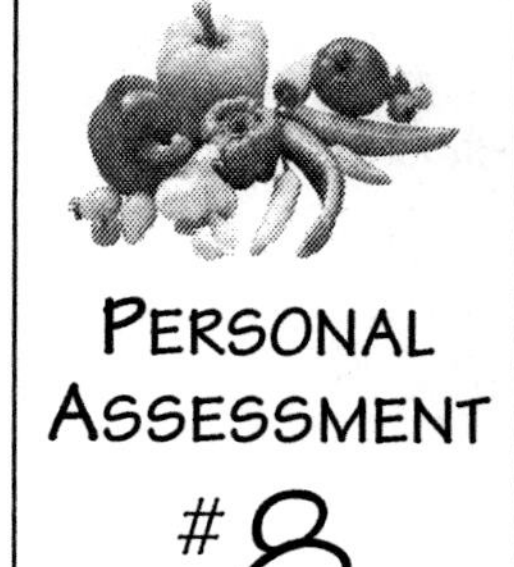

PERSONAL ASSESSMENT #8

Go to the following excellent CSPI site to check your answers to the following yes/no questions: http://www.cspinet.org/nah/11_00/index.html

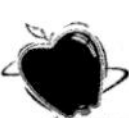

The Kitchen Sink	***The Big Chill***	***Grocery Know-How***
1. I wash my hands with soap or dishwashing liquid both *before* and *after* I handle food. ________	1. I keep a thermometer in my refrigerator and make sure that the temperature stays at 40°F or less. ________	1. I check "sell by" or "use by" dates on perishable foods before I buy them, and again before I use them. ________
2. I have a separate sponge only for wiping up spills from raw meat, poultry, seafood, and eggs. ________	2. If refrigerated meat, fish, or poultry smells okay, it's safe to eat. ________	2. I make sure to use any cracked eggs before the others. ________
3. I sometimes use my dish towel to wipe my hands while I'm cooking. ________	3. I give the inside of my refrigerator a thorough, warm soapy wash every month. ________	3. I cook or freeze steaks and chops within 3 or 4 days of purchase, fish within 24 to 36 hours of purchase, and poultry or ground meat within 1 or 2 days of purchase. ________
4. Plastic cutting boards are less likely to spread bacteria than wooden cutting boards. ________	4. I always defrost frozen meat, seafood, or poultry in the sink, so I can rinse the thawed juices right down the drain. ________	4. Dairy products need to be pasteurized, but fruit juices don't. ________
5. I give my fresh produce a good, warm soak in the sink before I use it. ________	5. If I'm using meat, poultry, or fish that has been frozen, I make sure to cook it the same day I defrost it. ________	5. It's okay to buy food in dented cans. ________

(continued)

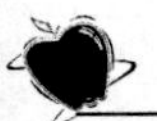

Clean-Up	What's Cookin'?
1. I wrap and refrigerate leftovers as soon as possible, and always within 2 hours. ______	1. I test to see whether poultry is done by piercing the skin of a leg or thigh. If the juices run pink, the bird needs more cooking. If the juices are clear, it's done. ______
2. I eat, freeze, or toss leftovers within a week. ______	2. Hamburgers and meat loaf are safe to eat if they're not pink in the middle. ______
3. I note the date and contents of leftovers on the container in which I store them. ______	3. When I serve cooked meat, eggs, seafood, or poultry, I use clean platters and utensils, not the ones I used when the food was raw or while it was cooking. ______
4. I clean my sponges at least once a week. ______	4. It's okay to baste meat, seafood, or poultry with its marinade as it's cooking. ______
5. After every meal that was prepared using raw meat, seafood, poultry, or eggs, I wash my counters and work surfaces with hot, soapy water. ______	5. It's okay to let my kids eat cold hot dogs right out of the package. ______

This quiz was devised by Diana Birkett and Mimi Harrison, with help from CSPI's Lucy Alderton and Caroline Smith DeWaal, and Jack Guzewich of the U.S. Food and Drug Administration.

Name ______________________________ Date ______________

Food Label Savvy

PERSONAL ASSESSMENT #9

Look at a **favorite food** label to analyze its nutritional value.

Answer the following for *1 serving*:

1. *Name* of product ______________
2. Total *Calories* per serving ______________
3. Number of *servings* per container ______________
4. The *largest* ingredient by weight ______________

Look at the **carbohydrate** section:

5. Number of total *carbohydrate* grams ______________
6. Number of *sugar* grams ______________
7. *% or ratio* of sugar to total carbs (Should be no more than 1/4–1/3) ______________
8. *Type* of sugar (brown rice syrup, molasses, sucrose) ______________
9. Total grams of *fiber* ______________
10. Any *descriptive term* for fiber? (good source = 2.5–4.9, high = 5.0+) ______________
11. *% carbs* of total Calories (grams × 4 divided by total Calories) ______________

Look at the **protein**:

12. Number of total *protein* grams ______________
13. Categorize protein *source* (plant or animal?) ______________
14. Describe protein gram *amount* ______________

Not a source	0 grams
Low source	.5–2 grams
Good source	2.5–5 grams
High source	Over 5 grams

15. *% Protein* of total Calories (grams × 4 divided by total Calories) ______________

Look at the **fat** section:

16. Number of total *fat* grams ____________

17. Number of *saturated fat* grams ____________

18. *Source* of fat (see ingredient list) ____________

19. Any *hydrogenated or trans fats*? ____________

20. Is product *low fat*? (3 grams or less per serving) ____________

21. *% fat* of total Calories (fat Calories divided by total Calories) ____________

Look at the **sodium:**

22. Total milligrams of *sodium* ____________

23. Is this product *low* in sodium? (Less than 140 mg) ____________

Look at the **vitamins and minerals**:

24. List any "*good or excellent source*" nutrients. ____________

____

____

____

25. Is your product rich in **phytonutrients**? (Why or why not?) ____________

26. Rank the product according to the following chart:
(remember quality of ingredients, such as organic, no additives, etc.) ____________

Foundation food	Good food to offer regularly/daily
Sometimes food	Food to offer a few times per week
*Seldom food	Food to offer very little, if at all

*Some foods may be "never" foods because they are not part of one's culture or beliefs or because one may have an allergy or intolerance to them.

Name ____________________ Date ____________

Carbo-Loading Calcs

Calculating Your Needs for an Endurance Event

PERSONAL ASSESSMENT #10

Record your weight in pounds ____________

Record your weight in kilograms ____________

3–5 days prior to the endurance event:

8–10 grams of carbohydrates per kilogram of body weight

Your grams of carbs per day ____________

Preevent meal 3–4 hours prior to event:

4–5 grams per kilogram of body weight

Your grams of carbs in preevent meal ____________

One hour before event:

1–2 grams per kilogram of body weight

Your grams of carbs 1 hour prior ____________

During event:

6–8 oz. of a 6% carb solution every 15–20 minutes

.6 grams carb per kilograms per hour

Your grams of carbs per hour during competition ____________

Postevent:

.6 grams per pound of body weight following exercise

Your grams of carbs 1 hour post ____________

(Remember 4:1 carb to protein ratio)

8–10 grams per kilogram in 24 hours following event

Your grams of carbs 24 hours post ____________

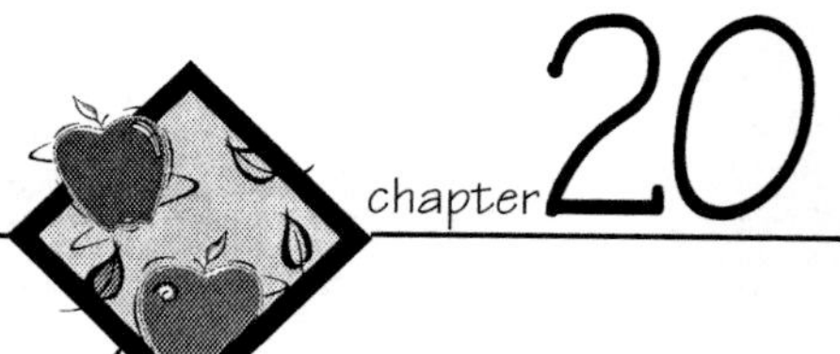

A Personalized Evaluation and Plan

Analyzing Your Diet and Setting Goals

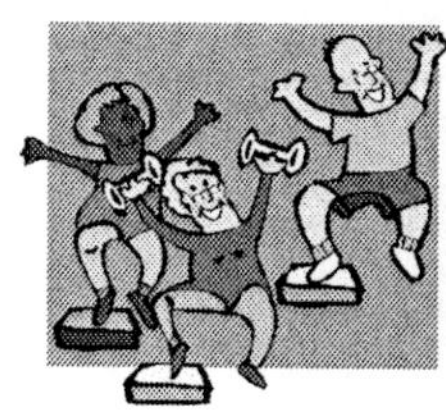

This final chapter allows you to take the information learned throughout the book along with the personal assessments and finally fully evaluate the nutritional quality and adequacy of your diet, then make suggestions for yourself on how to improve.

Evaluation of Your Diet

A. *CALORIES (Assessment #6)*

1. State how many calories you averaged for the 3 days. How did it compare to your needs?
2. Is this analysis more or less than your usual caloric intake? Why or why not?
3. State your height and current weight and body composition if you know it.
4. Have you been trying to gain or lose weight (fat) lately? How do you think your average calories influence this gain or loss? (Remember the pound-a-week rule.)

B. ***DISTRIBUTION OF CALORIES—See pie chart on printouts***

Note: It is recommended that your kcal be distributed as follows *(ONLY if your kcal are 100% of the RDA)*:

10%–15%	Protein (USE YOUR PROTEIN ASSESSMENT)
30% or less	Fat (ARE YOU UNDER 65 GRAMS/DAY? ARE YOU 20%?)
55% or more	Carbohydrates (DO YOU MEET YOUR CALCULATED NEEDS?)

1. **Protein: (Assessment #4, chapter 6)**
   State your % kcal from protein and answer one of the following statements. Then state whether your proteins are very lean, lean, medium fat, or high fat. Are they mainly plant or animal? Do you eat at least two plant protein sources daily?
   - If your grams fell short, suggest specific foods that would improve your protein intake.
   - If your grams were higher than your protein assignment calculation, how could you decrease your protein intake?
   - If your grams were within 15 grams of your calculation, explain how your diet stays at this recommended level. Caution: Listing all high-protein foods would indicate an excess.

2. **Carbohydrate: (Assessment #2, chapter 4)**
   State your % kcalories from carbs and answer one of the following statements. Be sure to note differences between complex, simple, refined, and unrefined carbs in your diet—not definitions of these terms. State whether or not you consume at least six servings daily of whole grains or starchy vegetables.
   - If your % kcal from carbs was lower than or equal to 55%, suggest specific foods that would improve your carbohydrate intake.
   - If your % kcal from carbs was greater than 55%, what foods contributed?

3. **Fat: (Assessment #3, chapter 5)**
   State your % kcal from fat and answer one of the following statements. (Explain your percent of poly, mono, and saturated fats. Are they each below 10% of total kcal? Is your saturated fat the lowest? Did you consume hydrogenated or trans fats?)
   - If your % kcal from fat exceeded or equaled 30%, describe changes in portion sizes or substitutions that will lower your fat intake.
   - If your % kcal from fat were less than 30% and 65 grams (preferably 20%), name specific foods that you do or don't eat that are responsible for your % kcal from fat.

4. **Alcohol**
   State whether you consumed alcohol and if so, what percentage of your Calories it represented. Do you feel this is a healthy or unhealthy amount consumed? How does it affect your overall diet?

C. *CHOLESTEROL (Assessment #3, chapter 5)*

1. State the mg of cholesterol that you consumed and answer one of the following questions.
   - If your diet exceeded 300 mg of cholesterol per day, suggest food changes that you could make to lower your cholesterol intake.
   - If your diet did not exceed 300 mg of cholesterol, name specific foods that you do or don't eat that are responsible for your cholesterol intake. **Remember that you do not need any cholesterol.**

D. *SODIUM (ALSO DO YOU HAVE A 1:1 SODIUM TO CALORIE RATIO?)*

1. State the mg of sodium that you consumed and answer one of the following statements.
   - If your sodium intake exceeded your profile maximum, suggest specific changes that you could make to lower your sodium intake.
   - If your diet contained less than your profile maximum mg of sodium, name specific foods that you do or don't eat that help keep your diet low in sodium.

E. *FIBER (Assessment #2, chapter 4)*

1. State the grams of fiber in your diet and answer one of the following statements. If you consumed more than 2000 Calories, figure fiber needs to be 10–15 extra grams for every 1000 Calories over 2000 Calories.
   - If your fiber intake was below 25 grams, suggest specific changes that you could make to improve your fiber intake.
   - If your fiber intake was greater then 25 grams, describe which foods helped you reach this level of fiber intake.

F. *VITAMINS (Assessment #5, chapter 8)*

These are the vitamins listed on the printout:

A C D E K B_1 B_2 Niacin B_6 Folate B_{12}

Answer one of the following statements:

1. List the vitamins you are deficient in (less than 100% of the RDA). For *each* deficient vitamin, suggest foods that will improve the intake of that vitamin. (MAKE SURE SUGGESTIONS ARE CONSISTENT W/MACRONUTRIENT GOALS!)
2. If you were not deficient in *any* vitamins, give specific examples of why your diet is able to meet the RDA recommendations.

G. *MINERALS (Assessment #5, chapter 8) (SODIUM ALREADY DISCUSSED.)*

These are the minerals listed on the printout:

Calcium Iron Magnesium Phosphorus Potassium Zinc

Answer one of the statements below:

1. List the minerals you are deficient in (less than 100% RDA). For *each* deficient mineral, suggest specific foods that will improve your intake of that mineral. (MAKE SURE SUGGESTIONS ARE CONSISTENT WITH MACRONUTRIENT GOALS!)
2. If you are not deficient in *any* minerals, give specific examples of why your diet is able to meet the RDA recommendations.

H. ***WATER (chapter 17)***

1. State the amount of water from the average printouts that you consumed daily.
2. Is this adequate for your personal needs? Why or why not?

I. ***CAFFEINE (chapter 16)***

1. State the amount of caffeine from the printouts that you consumed.
2. How do you feel about your caffeine consumption?

J. ***EXERCISE (Personal Assessment #7)***

1. Do you exercise aerobically at least three times a week?
2. List the types of flexibility, muscular endurance, and strength and aerobic exercises that you regularly do.

K. ***NUTRIENT SUPPLEMENTS***

1. Do you now take any nutrient supplements or have you taken them in the recent past?
2. *If you do* take supplements, indicate the types that you take and the frequency. (Use the information from supplement labels to indicate the amounts of the various ingredients.)
3. *If you do* take supplements, look at the computer printout for the 3-day average and indicate which nutrient supplements are probably unnecessary.

L. ***QUALITY AND PHYTONUTRIENTS (Assessment #5, chapter 8)***

Look at the color in your diet. List the foods that you ate in your 3 days from each color of the dietary color wheel which are rich in phytonutrients that prevent disease: Write "None" if you do not have a fruit or vegetable in a particular category.

Red ____________ ____________ ____________

Red (Blue)-Purple ____________ ____________ ____________

Orange ____________ ____________ ____________

Orange-Yellow ____________ ____________ ____________

Yellow-Green ____________ ____________ ____________

Green ____________ ____________ ____________

White Green ____________ ____________ ____________

M. ***OVERALL ADEQUACY OF DIET***

Select one of the following categories for your diet and describe why your diet fits into this category and any general changes that you need to make.

1. *Healthy and adequate*—meets 100% of all vitamin, mineral, protein, carbs, phytonutrients, and fiber requirements while staying low in fat, cholesterol, and sodium.
2. *Marginally okay*—meets almost 100% of all vitamin, mineral, protein, carbs, phytonutrients, and fiber requirements while staying low in fat, cholesterol, and sodium.
3. *Needs improvement*—meets only 50%–90% of most of the requirements and has some excesses of fat, cholesterol, and sodium.
4. *Dangerously inadequate*—meets less than 50% of most requirements and has many excesses of fat, cholesterol, and sodium.

N. GOALS FOR LIFESTYLE CHANGE

State your overall lifestyle goals for change, both exercise and nutrition related. Who will help you make changes? How will you accomplish your goals? How will you get feedback?

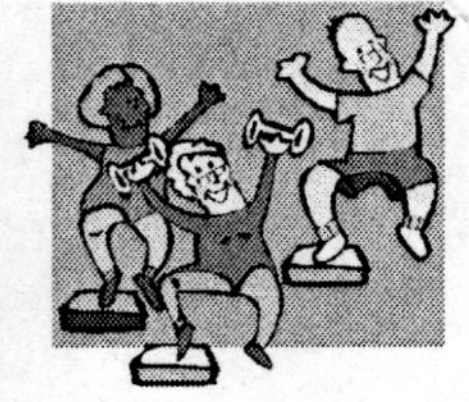

Now you are ready to begin implementing your Practical Nutrition for a Fit Life! Good luck!